MILADY® STANDARD

SHAVING

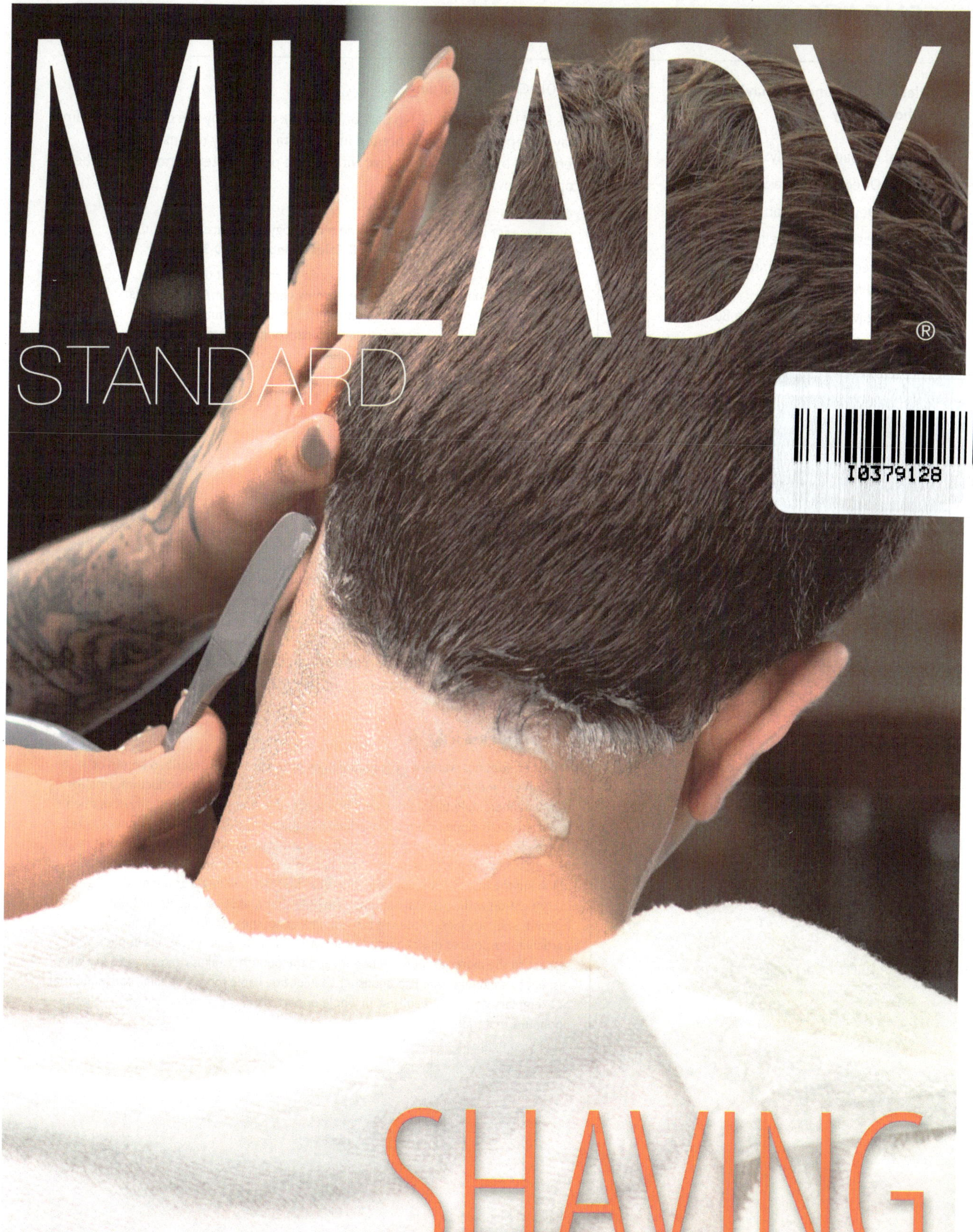

CENGAGE

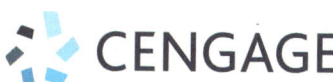

Australia • Brazil • Canada • Mexico • Singapore • United Kingdom • United States

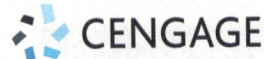

Title: Milady Standard Shaving
Author: Milady

General Manager, Milady: Sandra Bruce
Product Director: Corina Santoro
Content Developer: Sarah Prediletto
Product Assistant: Michelle Whitehead
Senior Director of Sales and Marketing: Gerard McAvey
Marketing Manager: Elizabeth Bushey
Senior Content Project Manager: Nina Tucciarelli
Art Director: Angela Sheehan
Text Designer: Angela Sheehan
Cover Designer: Angela Sheehan
Cover Image: Joseph and Yuki Paradiso

© 2018 Cengage Learning, Inc.

ALL RIGHTS RESERVED. No part of this work covered by the copyright herein may be reproduced or distributed in any form or by any means, except as permitted by U.S. copyright law, without the prior written permission of the copyright owner.

> For product information and technology assistance, contact us at
> **Cengage Customer & Sales Support, 1-800-354-9706**
> For permission to use material from this text or product,
> submit all requests online at **www.cengage.com/permissions.**
> Further permissions questions can be e-mailed to
> **permissionrequest@cengage.com**

Library of Congress Control Number: 2014950279

ISBN: 978-1-337-62045-1

Cengage
200 Pier 4 Boulevard
Boston, MA 02210
USA

Cengage is a leading provider of customized learning solutions with employees residing in nearly 40 different countries and sales in more than 125 countries around the world. Find your local representative at **www.cengage.com**.

To learn more about Cengage platforms and services, register or access your online learning solution, or purchase materials for your course, visit **www.cengage.com**.

Notice to the Reader

Publisher does not warrant or guarantee any of the products described herein or perform any independent analysis in connection with any of the product information contained herein. Publisher does not assume, and expressly disclaims, any obligation to obtain and include information other than that provided to it by the manufacturer. The reader is expressly warned to consider and adopt all safety precautions that might be indicated by the activities described herein and to avoid all potential hazards. By following the instructions contained herein, the reader willingly assumes all risks in connection with such instructions. The publisher makes no representations or warranties of any kind, including but not limited to, the warranties of fitness for particular purpose or merchantability, nor are any such representations implied with respect to the material set forth herein, and the publisher takes no responsibility with respect to such material. The publisher shall not be liable for any special, consequential, or exemplary damages resulting, in whole or part, from the readers' use of, or reliance upon, this material.

Printed at CLDPC, USA, 06-24

BRIEF CONTENTS AND INTRODUCTION

Contents

Know about Straight Razors 2

Show How to Hold a Straight Razor 3

Understand the Fundamentals of Shaving 10

Understand Facial-Hair Design 21

Review Shaving-Related Infection Control and Safety Precautions 24

Procedures 1 to 12 26–68

Activities 71

Test Preparation 81

Milady Standard Shaving

Milady Standard Shaving is your comprehensive guide to learning the art of straight razor shaving. This supplement provides an overview of the tools and implements involved, the theory of shaving, and step-by-step instructions for every procedure.

In addition to the traditional book content, we have also included activities and a practice test to help you master the content. The Activities section contains fill-in-the-blank, true or false, multiple choice, essay, short answer, labeling, and matching activities. The Test Preparation is multiple choice to help to prepare you for your licensure exam.

Milady Standard Shaving, combined with the guidance of your instructor, will prepare you for your licensure examination and ensure that you graduate with the skill set and confidence to shave throughout your career.

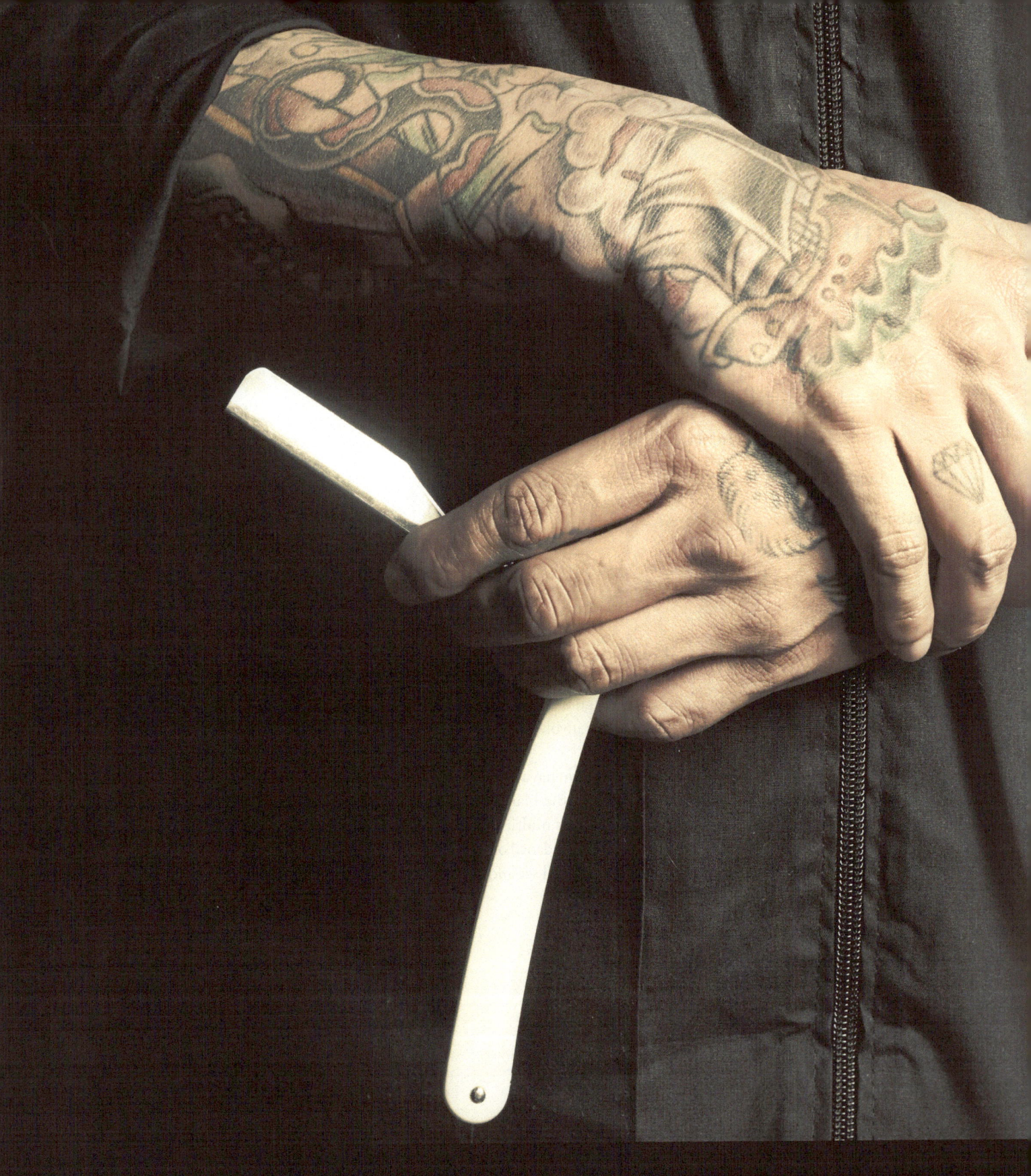

MILADY STANDARD SHAVING

LEARNING OBJECTIVES

After completing this section, you will be able to:

LO 1
Name two types of straight razors.

LO 2
Identify the different parts of a straight razor.

LO 3
Show how to hold a straight razor for shaving, honing, and stropping.

LO 4
Show how to hold a straight razor for haircutting.

LO 5
Describe the functions of hones and strops.

LO 6
Show how to hone and strop a conventional blade straight razor.

LO 7
List basic guidelines for shaving a client.

LO 8
Identify the 14 shaving areas of the face.

LO 9
Explain what you need to know about razor positions and strokes to perform a shave safely and effectively.

LO 10
Describe the differences between various facial-hair designs.

LO 11
Discuss infection control and safety precautions associated with shaving.

LO 12
Demonstrate how to handle a straight razor safely.

LO 13
Demonstrate the freehand, backhand, reverse-freehand and reverse-backhand positions and strokes.

LO 14
Demonstrate a shave service.

LO 15
Demonstrate a neck shave.

LO 16
Demonstrate a mustache trim.

LO 17
Demonstrate cutting in beard designs.

Know about Straight Razors

After reading this section, you will be able to:

 Name two types of straight razors.

 Identify the different parts of a straight razor.

As the sharpest and closest cutting tool, razors are used for facial shaves, head shaves, neck shaves, finish work around the sideburn and behind-the-ear areas, and haircutting. The razor of choice for professional shaving is the straight razor; safety razors are not used to perform professional shaving services in the salon.

The two types of straight razors used in shaving are the **changeable-blade straight razor** (CHAYNJE-able BLAYD STRAYT RAY-zor) and the **conventional straight razor** (kun-VEN-shun-ul STRAYT RAY-zor). Both may be purchased with a razor guard for use in razor-cutting the hair.

Selecting the right kind of razor is a matter of personal choice. The best guides for buying high-quality razors are as follows:

- Consult with a reliable company representative or salesperson who can recommend the type of razor best suited to your work.
- Consult with more experienced professionals about which razors they have found best for shaving and haircutting.
- Experiment with a variety of razors to determine the style and type most comfortable for you based on the service to be performed. For example, you may prefer a longer blade razor when performing a facial shave and a shorter blade razor for arching around the ears during a haircut.
- Avoid judging a razor simply on color or design. Neither one of these characteristics provides a true indication of the razor's caliber as a cutting tool.

IDENTIFY THE PARTS OF A STRAIGHT RAZOR

The structural parts of conventional and changeable-blade straight razors are basically the same except in the blade area; the conventional razor has a blade and the changeable-blade razor has a blade holder for the blade. Therefore, the structural parts of a straight razor are the head, back, shoulder, tang, shank, heel, edge, point, blade or blade holder, pivot, and handle (**Figure 1**).

DESCRIBE CHANGEABLE-BLADE STRAIGHT RAZORS

The changeable- (or disposable-) blade straight razor closely resembles a conventional straight razor in its overall design. This type of razor tends to be used almost exclusively in the professional shaving because its disposable blade eliminates honing and stropping, saves time, and helps to maintain infection control standards (**Figure 2**).

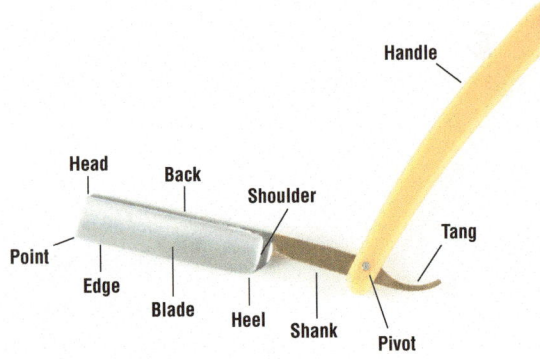

figure 1
Parts of a razor.

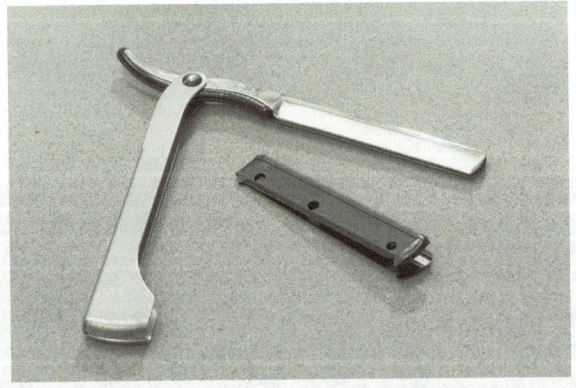

figure 2
Changeable-blade razor.

Razor Shapers

There are a variety of razor shapers (also known as hair shapers) available on the market today. One style made of lightweight metal with a pivot and open-handle construction leaves the majority of the blade visible (**Figure 3**). This type of razor is not recommended for facial shaving because the blade size and shape can make it challenging to safely shave smaller areas, such as above the upper lip. Other hair shaper designs do not have a pivot and consist of a stationary handle with a finger rest (**Figure 4**). Both styles use a changeable-blade system and come with a guard.

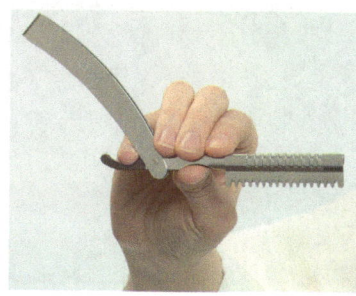

figure 3
Razor shaper.

FOLLOW MANUFACTURER'S DIRECTIONS FOR CHANGING THE BLADE

There are several changeable-razor models available and each will have its own design for holding the blade in place; therefore, the method for replacing the blade will vary depending on the model.

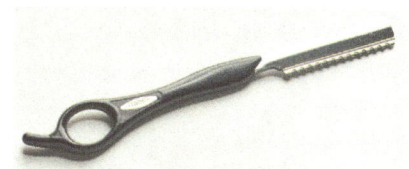

figure 4
Hair razor.

Show How to Hold a Straight Razor

After reading this section, you will be able to:

- **LO 3** Show how to hold a straight razor for shaving, honing, and stropping.
- **LO 4** Show how to hold a straight razor for haircutting.
- **LO 5** Describe the functions of hones and strops.
- **LO 6** Show how to hone and strop a conventional blade straight razor.

HOLDING THE STRAIGHT RAZOR

How you hold the straight razor will depend on the procedure to be performed, the type of razor you use, and the positioning that gives you the most control of the razor. Refer to **Figures 5 to 9** and the following section to consider several holding techniques.

- **Shaving:** The ball of the thumb and first two fingers are positioned on the flat side of the shanks with the handle pivoted up to allow the little finger to rest on the tang. This positions the razor at a better angle while providing more control over the razor (**Figure 5**).

- **Honing and stropping:** The ball of the thumb and first two fingers are positioned on the flat sides of the shank with the handle in a straight position (**Figure 6**).

- **Haircutting:** The ball of the thumb supports the razor at the bottom of the shank and the little finger rests on the tang, with the first two or three fingers at the top of the shank (**Figure 7**). Or, the razor handle is in a straightened position with the thumb and first two fingers almost touching at the shank (**Figure 8**).

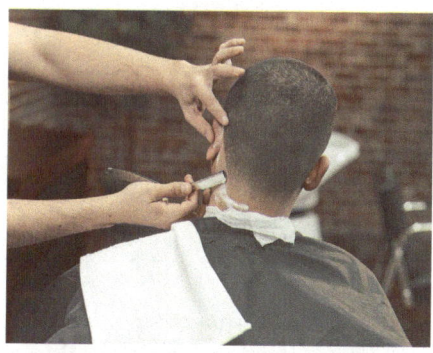

figure 5
Stroke with razor.

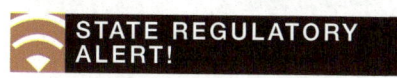

STATE REGULATORY ALERT!

Some state boards prohibit the use of conventional straight razors. Be sure to check the rules and regulations in your state before purchase or use.

MILADY STANDARD SHAVING   3

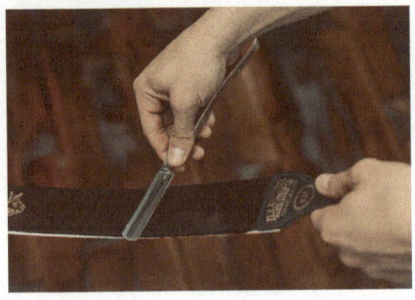
figure 6
Razor strop.

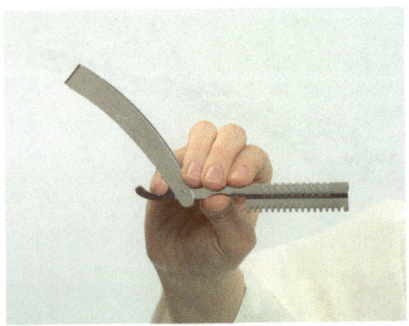
figure 7
Holding the razor shaper properly.

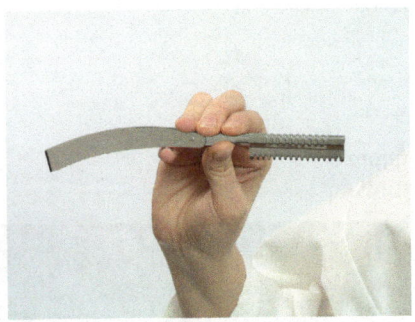
figure 8
Alternate method of holding the razor shaper.

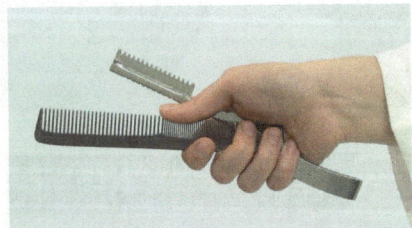
figure 9
Palming the razor and comb.

- Holding the comb and razor: To palm the razor for hair combing, simply roll the razor into your hand with the blade facing away from the comb. Hold the comb between the thumb and first two fingers (Figure 9). Keep a firm grip on the razor to prevent it from slipping and cutting your hand during combing.

LEARN ABOUT CONVENTIONAL STRAIGHT RAZORS

The conventional straight razor requires honing and stropping to maintain its cutting edge. This razor is composed of a hardened steel blade attached to a handle by means of a pivot. The handle may be constructed of hard rubber, plastic, metal, or new polymer materials.

Consider Razor Quality

In order to determine the quality of a razor, you must consider the following factors: razor balance, temper, grind, finish, size, and style.

Razor Balance

Razor balance refers to the weight and length of the blade relative to that of the handle. A straight razor is properly balanced when the weight of the blade and handle are equal. Proper balance of the razor allows for greater ease and safety in handling the razor during shaving. Opening the razor and resting it on the index finger at the pivot will test the balance of the razor. If the head of the razor moves up or down, the razor is not well balanced.

Razor Temper

Tempering the razor refers to a special heat treatment included in the manufacturing process. When a razor is properly tempered, it acquires the degree of hardness required for a good cutting edge. Razors can be purchased with a hard, soft, or medium temper. The professional should select the temper that produces the most satisfactory shaving results. While hard-tempered razors will hold an edge longer, they are difficult to sharpen; conversely, soft-tempered razors are easier to sharpen, but the sharp edge does not last long. For those reasons, many professionals prefer a medium-tempered razor.

Razor Grind

The grind of a razor is the shape of the blade after it has been ground. There are two general types: the concave grind and the wedge grind (Figure 10).

- *Concave grind:* The concave grind (often referred to as the hollow ground) is available in full concave, one-half concave, and one-quarter concave forms. The back and edge of the razor looks hollow, being slightly thicker between the hollow part and the extreme edge. Many professionals prefer the hollow-ground razor since the resistance of a beard can be felt more easily and alerts the professional to check the sharpness of the cutting edge. Although the one-half and one-quarter concave grinds are less hollow than the full concave, the outside dimensions of the blade appear the same.
- *Wedge grind:* The wedge grind is neither hollow nor concave. Both sides of the blade form a sharp angle at the extreme edge of the razor. Most older razors were made with a wedge grind. Although learning how to sharpen a wedge grind may be a challenge, once mastered, this grind produces an excellent shave. It is especially preferred for men with coarse, heavy beards.

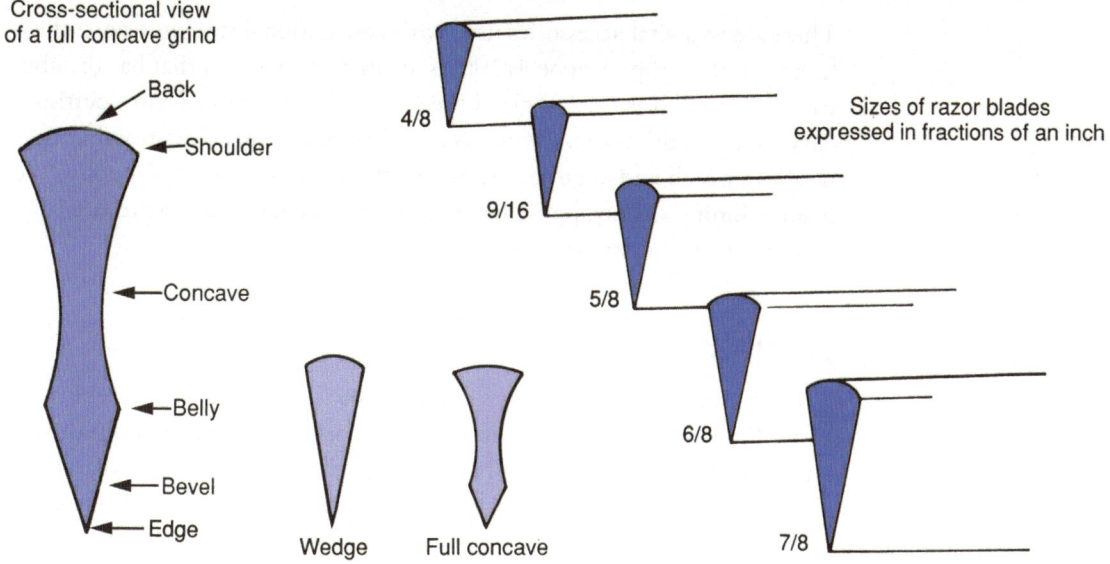

figure 10
Razor grinds.

Razor Finish
The finish of a razor is the polish of its surface. This finish may be plain, crocus (polished steel), or plated with nickel or silver. Of these types, the crocus finish is usually the choice of the discriminating professional. Although the crocus finish is more costly, it lasts longer and does not rust as easily as other finishes. Metal-plated razors are undesirable because the finish wears off quickly and may hide poor-quality steel.

Razor Size
The size of the razor is measured by the length and width of the blade. The width of the razor is measured either in eighths or sixteenths of an inch, such as 4/8 inches, 5/8 inches, 6/8 inches, 7/8 inches, and 9/16 inches. Two of the most common sizes are the 5/8 inches and 9/16 inches, the 5/8 inches being the more popular.

Razor Style
The style of a razor indicates its shape and design. Modern razors have such features as a back and edge that are straight and parallel to each other; a round heel; a square point; and a flat or slightly round handle. To avoid scratching the skin, the professional usually rounds off the square point of the razor slightly by drawing the point of the razor along the edge of the hone.

Razor Care
Razors will maintain their quality if care is taken to prevent corrosion of the extremely fine edge. After use, a razor should be cleaned, stropped, and a little oil applied to the cutting edge. Be careful not to drop the razor as doing so may damage the blade. When closing the razor, be careful that the cutting edge does not strike the handle. If the cutting edge strikes the handle when closing the razor, it may indicate that the handle is warped or that the pivot is too tightly riveted. The tool kit should include several high-grade razors so that a damaged razor can be replaced immediately.

IDENTIFY ACCESSORIES USED WITH CONVENTIONAL STRAIGHT RAZORS

There are two vital accessories used with conventional straight razors: the hone and the strop. A **hone** (HOHN) is an abrasive material that has the ability to cut steel. It is used to grind the steel and impart an effective cutting edge to the razor's blade. A **strop** is a leather and canvas accessory that is used to smooth and align the cutting teeth of the razor edge and polish the blade. Honing and stropping techniques must be mastered to prepare a conventional straight razor for shaving.

HONES

There are various types of hones available for the purpose of sharpening razors. Hones are manufactured in a rectangular block shape, without or with an attached handle, for ease of blade placement on the surface. Since the abrasive material of the hone is harder than steel, it will cut or file the edge on the blade of the razor.

Students should practice with a slow-cutting hone, while experienced practitioners generally use a faster-cutting hone.

There are three main types of hones: natural, synthetic, and combination.

- Natural hones are cut from natural rock formations. The two types of natural hones are the water hone and the Belgium hone. These hones have a slow cutting action that can produce a fine, long-lasting edge when used with water or shaving lather to lubricate the stone before sharpening.
- Synthetic hones, such as the carborundum hone, are manufactured products. These hones cut faster than water hones, producing a keen cutting edge in less time and may be used wet or dry, although you need to take care not to over-hone the razor.
- Combination hones consist of both a water hone and a synthetic hone. The synthetic side is used first to develop a good cutting edge and the natural side is used to produce a fine finished edge.

Choosing a Hone

When selecting a hone, remember that the finer the abrasive, the slower its action. Many professionals use combination hones; however, it is advisable to be familiar with the other types of hones and to understand the benefits of each. The type of steel in the razor also makes some difference as to whether a good edge can be obtained with a particular type of hone. Be guided by your instructor, personal experimentation with different hones, and razor manufacturer's recommendations.

Care of Hones

Always clean the hone before use. Use water and a pumice stone to remove the tiny steel particles that accumulate on the surface of the hone. If a new hone is very rough, the same method can be used to work it into shape.

When wet honing is done, always wipe the hone dry after use. This aids the cleaning process and also wipes away the particles of steel that adhere to the cutting surface. Always disinfect the hone according to the manufacturer's directions.

Honing Guidelines

Review the following guidelines before practicing the honing techniques in Procedure 1.

- Position the index finger along the top of the shank to ensure even pressure against the blade while honing.
- Make sure your fingertips do not project above the edge of the hone to avoid injury.
- The razor is stroked *edge-first* diagonally across the hone. This produces teeth with a cutting edge.
- The edge blade should be kept flat on the hone, with no rocking or lifting from the surface.
- Stroke the blade with equal pressure from heel to point and from side to side.
- An equal number of strokes should be made on both sides of the blade.
- The angle at which the blade is stroked must be the same for both of its sides.
- As the blade edge is sharpened, gradually lighten the pressure and test frequently.
- The number of strokes required in honing depends on the condition of the razor's edge.

Testing a Honed Blade

A honed blade is tested by lightly passing it over a thumbnail moistened with water or lather (**Figure 11**). You should feel one of the following sensations as the blade edge passes over your nail:

- A keen edge has fine teeth and tends to dig into the nail with a smooth, steady grip.
- A blunt or dull razor edge passes over the nail smoothly without any cutting power.
- A coarse razor edge digs into the nail with a jerky feeling.
- A coarse or over-honed edge has large teeth that stick to the nail and produce a harsh, grating sound.
- A nick in the razor produces the feeling of a slight gap or unevenness when drawn across the nail.

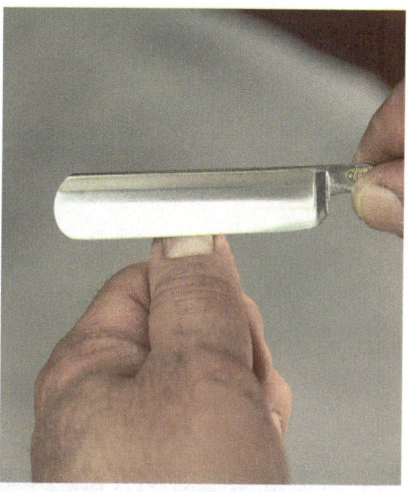

figure 11
Testing a honed razor.

> **CAUTION**
> This testing technique requires a great deal of practice and experience. Be very cautious of the amount of pressure and speed with which the test is performed. Touch the razor's edge lightly, and note the sensation you feel. A dull edge does not produce a drawing sensation. A proper cutting edge will have a sharp drawing sensation. If the razor's edge yields a smooth feeling upon testing, finish it again on the canvas strop, followed by a few more strokes on the leather strop.

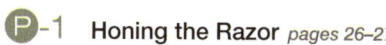 **P-1   Honing the Razor** *pages 26–27*

STROPS

Unlike hones, which are designed to grind the edge of a razor into a sharp cutting edge, strops are used to remove small metal particles from the blade,

> **DID YOU KNOW?**
> Finer-quality strops are usually "broken in" by the manufacturer, thereby requiring less breaking in and preparation by the professional.

to smooth the edge, and to polish the razor. A good strop is made of durable and flexible material with the proper thickness and texture and shows a smooth, finished surface. Some professionals like a thin strop; others prefer a thick, heavy strop.

Strops are generally classified as leather or canvas. Cowhide and horsehide are the most common leathers used to manufacture a strop. The four types of strops covered in this section are the combination, canvas, Russian, and shell strops.

- The combination strop is the type of strop most commonly used by professionals because it is an all-in-one accessory for preparing the razor after honing. This strop is actually made of two strops—a canvas strop and a leather strop—that have been riveted together at the attachment end of the strop.

- A **canvas strop** (can-viss strohp), or the canvas side of a combination strop, should be made of high-quality linen or silk, woven into a fine or coarse texture. A fine-textured canvas strop is desirable for removing any metal burrs or imbrications that remain after honing. To obtain the best results, a new canvas strop should be thoroughly broken in. Consult manufacturer's instructions for recommended products and directions to prepare and maintain a canvas strop.

- The **Russian strop** (RUSH-an strohp) was originally imported from Russia and still bears the name even though it may be manufactured elsewhere. The name simply implies that the Russian method of tanning was used to prepare the leather. Russian strops are usually made from cowhide and are considered to be one of the best. Consult the manufacturer's instructions for recommended products and directions to prepare and maintain a Russian strop.

> **DID YOU KNOW?**
> If a strop is labeled "Russian shell strop," it indicates that the strop is made from the rump area of a horse and that the Russian tanning method was used in its manufacture.

- A **shell strop** is a high-quality strop taken from the muscular rump area of a horse. Although shell strops can be expensive, they are considered to be one of the best strops for professionals as they tend to remain smooth and require very little, if any, breaking in. As with other strops, consult the manufacturer's instructions for recommended products and directions to prepare and maintain your shell strop.

> **DID YOU KNOW?**
> The direction of the razor's edge used in stropping is the reverse of the direction used in honing.

Strop Dressing

Strop dressing cleans the leather strop, preserves its finish, and also improves its draw and sharpening qualities. Refer to the manufacturer's directions for proper application methods, timing in between applications, and follow-up procedures.

STROPPING THE RAZOR

From a technical standpoint, the razor may be stropped from the professional's hand toward the chair or from the chair to the hand. When performed correctly, both methods can achieve the same results; however, your state board may have a preferred method. Be sure to check the rules, regulations, and exam performance requirements in your state.

Stropping Guidelines

Review the following guidelines before practicing the stropping techniques in Procedure 2.

- The strop is attached to the arm of the chair by a closed clip.
- Hold the end of the strop firmly in your nondominant hand so it cannot sag and on a slight diagonal from the chair at a comfortable height.
- When holding the razor, the index finger is on the shank, the subsequent fingers are on the handle, and the thumb rests at the pivot. The index finger of your dominant hand should rest along the edge of the strop.
- The direction of the blade edge in stropping is the reverse of that used in honing; therefore, the back of the razor will lead each stroke, rather than the blade edge.
- Stropping the razor requires being able to roll the razor on its back after completing a stroke to position it for the next one. With the thumb on the side of the shank closest to you and the first two fingers braced on the other side of the shank, use your thumb to roll the blade up and over for the next stroke.
- Strokes should be made in a single, slightly diagonal stroke against the strop, with even pressure from the heel to the point of the razor.
- The blade edge needs to be flat against the surface to avoid cutting or nicking the strop.
- Bear down just enough to feel the razor draw against the strop.
- Do not worry about speed; a moderate pace is preferred.
- Strokes should be repeated as necessary to finish the razor edge.

> **CAUTION**
> When testing the razor's edge on the moistened tip of the thumb, a proper cutting edge will have a sharp drawing sensation. Use minimal pressure and speed to perform the test safely.

 P-2 Stropping the Razor *page 28*

Shaving and Facial-Hair Design

When performed correctly, a full facial shave, complete with hot towels, lotions, and massage, is one of the most relaxing, yet rejuvenating, services men can enjoy. And although safety and electric razors may have made it more convenient for men to shave at home, this self-service approach does not provide the preparation, relaxation, and finishing elements of a well-executed shave.

Your client can also benefit from mustache and beard trims being performed in the salon, since you are is better positioned and trained to create a more balanced and even facial-hair design.

> **CAUTION**
> It is critical that students read and study the entire shaving section before practicing a facial shave.

Understand the Fundamentals of Shaving

After reading this section, you will be able to:

LO 7 List basic guidelines for shaving a client.

LO 8 Identify the 14 shaving areas of the face.

LO 9 Explain what you need to know about razor positions and strokes to perform a shave safely and effectively.

The primary objective of shaving is to remove the visible part of facial and neck hair without causing irritation to the skin. A changeable-blade or conventional straight razor, hot towels, and warm lather are used in a professional shave.

Although there are general shaving principles that apply to all men, there are also exceptions that will require consideration. For example, the application of hot towels is a standard procedure in preparing the beard for shaving. However, some clients may not be able to tolerate a hot towel on their skin. Other individual characteristics such as hair texture, growth pattern, and product sensitivity are variables that must be considered before proceeding with the shave service.

CONSIDER BASIC GUIDELINES FOR SHAVING A CLIENT

There are some basic guidelines that you need to be aware of before shaving any client. These include some general dos and don'ts, characteristics of facial hair that need to be considered, and customer service concerns. Consider these important guidelines related to performing a shave service.

DOS AND DON'TS

- The client's skin must be analyzed before beginning the shave. Do not proceed with the service if the client has a skin infection or pustules. Doing so could spread the infection to other parts of the client's face or to you.
- The client's hair growth pattern must be analyzed before beginning the shave to identify grain changes and growth patterns in the beard.
- Do not use hot towels on skin that is chapped, blistered, thin, or sensitive.
- Do not perform a deep cleansing facial immediately after a shave as it may irritate or damage the skin.

- Be careful when shaving sensitive areas beneath the lower lip, on the lower part of the neck, and around the Adam's apple to avoid irritation or injury.

- Use pH-balanced fresheners or toners when stronger astringents are too harsh for sensitive skin.

- Heavy beard growth may require more thorough lathering and more hot-towel applications to prepare it for the shave.

- When a client wears a mustache, trim and shape it prior to the shave service to prepare it for finish work with the razor during the shave.

Hair Type Considerations

Curly facial hair requires special care because it grows in a looped direction as it grows out of the follicle; if not shaved correctly, it can bend back into the skin surface where it may cause ingrown hairs (pseudofolliculitis). Ingrown hairs are often the result of improper hair removal by a razor, tweezers, or trimmer. Improper hair removal includes excessively close shaving, shaving in the wrong direction, and/or excessive pressure with clippers, trimmers, or razors. Any of these methods can cause new hair to be trapped or pushed under the skin and if left untreated may result in infected bumps both on and under the skin surface (folliculitis). Sometimes, it may even initiate a keloid condition.

Hair Growth Considerations

You will need to analyze the direction and pattern of hair growth before beginning the shave to identify where the grain changes occur and to observe growth patterns that may influence the procedure.

- As hair emerges from the skin surface it flows in a particular direction. This direction of hair growth creates the *grain* of the hair. A *grain change* occurs when hair growing in one direction meets hair that is growing in a different or an opposite direction.

- Hair growth patterns are visible indicators of the direction of the hair as it emerges from the skin surface. Growth patterns determine hairline shapes and whether the hair lies down as it emerges from the skin or results in a whorl, cowlick, or other growth feature.

- The direction of hair growth determines the razor positions and strokes that need to be used to shave *with the grain* of the hair during the service.

While men's facial hair usually grows in the same direction in each of the 14 shaving areas, there are always exceptions. Occasionally, a section of the beard or neck hair will grow in a whorl pattern and may require the use of a different razor stroke than the stroke generally used in that particular shaving area. This is a perfectly acceptable practice when the growth pattern warrants the use of a different razor position or stroke.

Customer Satisfaction

While there are many reasons why a client may find fault with a shave procedure, the most common include

- dull or rough razors;
- unclean hands, towels, or drape;
- cold fingers;
- heavy touch;
- poorly heated towels (either too hot or too cold);
- poorly heated lather (either too hot or too cold);
- glaring overhead lights;
- unshaven hair patches;
- scraping the skin and close shaving;
- offensive body odor or foul breath of the professional.

> **CAUTION**
> Hones and strops are made of porous materials that can be cleaned, but not disinfected; therefore, a conventional straight razor must be cleaned and disinfected after the honing and stropping procedures before using it for a shave service.

IDENTIFY THE SHAVING AREAS OF THE FACE

There are 14 shaving areas of the face to be shaved during the *first-time-over* part of the service. These areas are shaved systematically and sequentially from one section to another using a specific razor position to shave *with the grain* in each area.

Refer to **Figures 12** through **17** and **Table 1** to review the 14 shaving areas of the face.

> **DID YOU KNOW?**
> Some states may require the use of protective gloves while shaving a client. Always check your state board regulations for rules related to shaving.

Shaving Areas for the Right-Handed Student

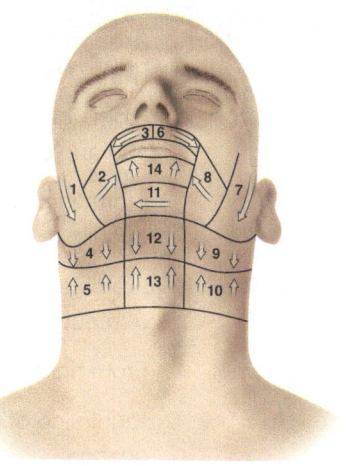

figure 12
Areas of the face for right-handed shaving: front.

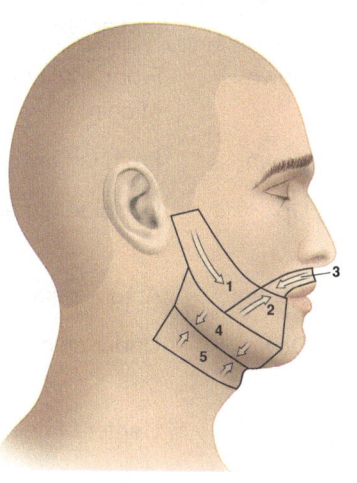

figure 13
Areas of the face for right-handed shaving: right side.

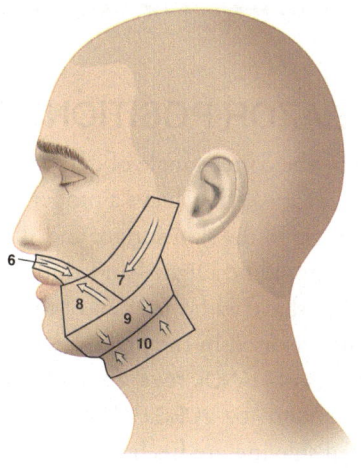

figure 14
Areas of the face for right-handed shaving: left side.

Shaving Areas for the Left-Handed Student

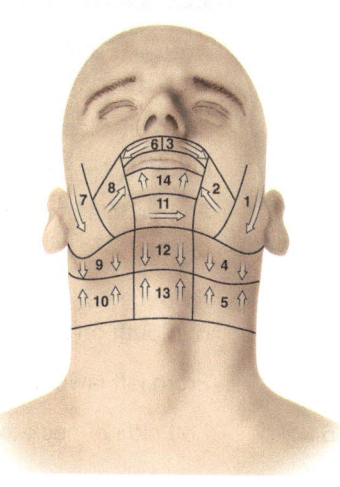

figure 15
Areas of the face for left-handed shaving: front.

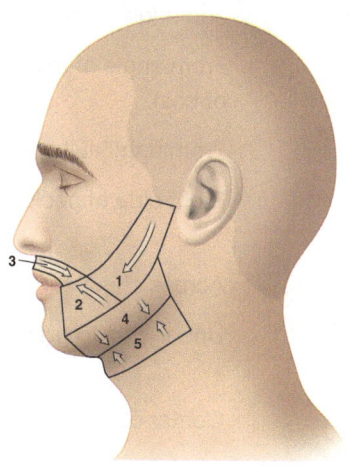

figure 16
Areas of the face for left-handed shaving: left side.

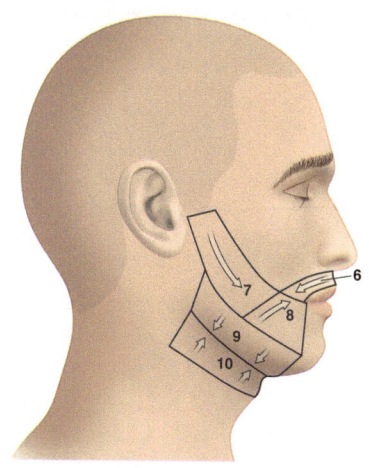

figure 17
Areas of the face for left-handed shaving: right side.

MILADY STANDARD SHAVING

table 1
SHAVING MOVEMENTS FOR LEFT-HANDED AND RIGHT-HANDED STUDENTS

Shaving Area	Area of Face for Left-Handed Student	Position and Stroke	Direction of Stroke	Area of Face for Right-Handed Student
1	From left sideburn toward jawbone and angle of mouth	Freehand	Down	From right sideburn toward jawbone and angle of mouth
2	From angle of mouth toward point of chin	Backhand	Down	From angle of mouth toward point of chin
3	From center of upper lip to corner of mouth on left side	Freehand	Down	From center of upper lip to corner of mouth on right side
4	From left jawbone to grain change	Freehand	Down	From right jawbone to grain change
5	Left side of neck to grain change	Reverse freehand	Up	Right side of neck up to grain change
6	From center of lip to corner of right side of mouth	Backhand	Down	From center of lip to corner of left side of mouth
7	From right sideburn toward jawbone and angle of mouth	Backhand	Down	From left sideburn toward jawbone and angle of mouth
8	From angle of mouth toward point of chin	Freehand	Down	From angle of mouth toward point of chin
9	From right jawbone to grain change	Backhand	Down	From left jawbone to grain change
10	Right side of neck to grain change	Reverse freehand	Up	Left side of neck to grain change
11	Across chin from right to left	Freehand	Across	Across chin from left to right
12	Under chin to grain change	Freehand or backhand	Down	Under chin to grain change
13	Center of neck to grain change	Reverse freehand	Up	Center of neck to grain change
14	Beneath lower lip	Reverse freehand	Up	Beneath lower lip

UNDERSTAND RAZOR POSITIONS AND STROKES

The term used to describe the correct angle of cutting with a razor is called the **cutting stroke** (KUT-ing STROHK). To achieve a proper cutting stroke, the razor is positioned at a slight angle to the skin surface and stroked with the point leading (Figure 18). This should be a light-handed forward gliding motion that is most often positioned to shave with the grain of the hair, not against it.

The four razor positions used in the practice of shaving are **freehand** (FREE-HAND), **backhand** (BAK-HAND), **reverse freehand** (ree-VURS FREE-HAND), and **reverse backhand** (ree-VURS BAK-HAND). The three positions and strokes used in facial shaving are freehand, backhand, and reverse freehand (see Figures 19 to 21).

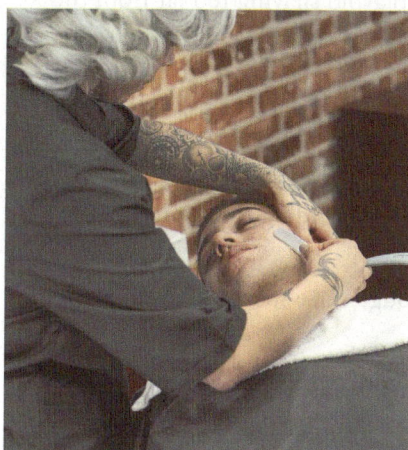

figure 18
Angle of cutting stroke (on skin).

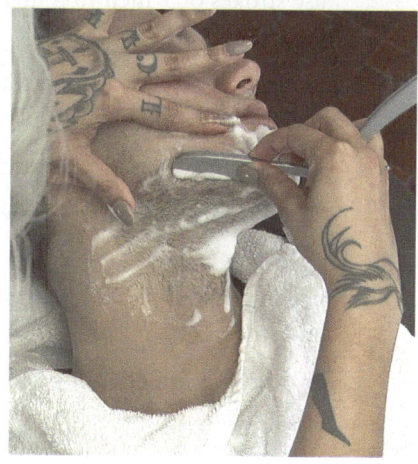

figure 19
Freehand position.

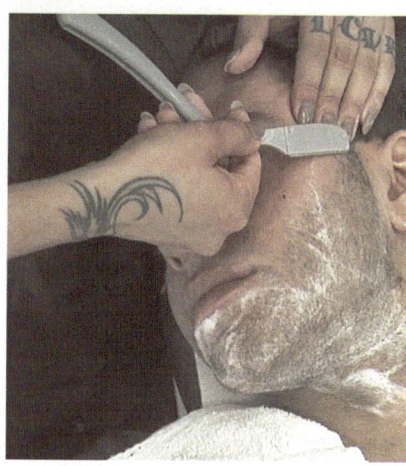

figure 20
Backhand position.

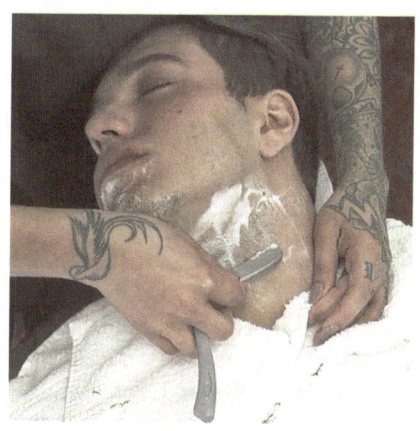

figure 21
Reverse-freehand position.

Position refers to the way the razor is held in the student hand to perform a stroke movement. For example, your instructor may direct you to "hold the razor in the freehand position" or "position the razor at about a 30-degree angle." The stroke is the actual movement of the razor as it is held in one of the four positions, for example, "a freehand stroke is used to shave area 1" or "use a gliding stroke toward you."

You will need to know and practice the following skills for each of the 14 shaving areas (refer to Procedures 3 and 4):

P-3 Handling a Straight Razor *pages 29–30*

P-4 Razor Position and Strokes Practice *pages 31–33*

- Where to use a particular razor position and stroke
- How to hold the razor for each position and stroke to
  - position the fingers, wrist, and elbow of the dominant hand in relation to the razor
  - position the opposite hand on the client's skin in relation to the razor
  - position your body in relation to the client to facilitate a razor position and stroke
- How to hold or stretch the skin to
  - find the balance between stretching the skin too much or too little
  - use the cushions of the fingertips to stretch the skin with the proper amount of pressure
  - use the thumb and second finger as the primary digits for stretching the skin
  - stretch different areas of the skin in the opposite direction that the razor will travel
- How to position and stroke the razor on the surface of the skin to
  - angle the razor about 30 degrees relative to the skin surface
  - use a forward gliding movement that leads with the point of the razor

- use the proper stroke length on different areas of the face
- use strokes of 1 inch to 3 inches to avoid shaving too far from the stretching point
- use shorter strokes around the mouth, over the ears, and in other tight areas
- develop a medium stroke speed to avoid very fast or very slow movements
- adjust the rate of speed of the stroke according to the area being shaved
- use smooth strokes that carry through once started without stopping and starting

• How to recognize growth patterns and the grain of the hair in different areas of the face to
- identify areas where the direction of hair growth changes
- use the appropriate razor position and stroke for the area to be shaved
- adjust stroke speed and pressure to accommodate the texture or density of the hair
- recognize use of the terms *with the grain*, *against the grain*, and *across the grain*

• How to work efficiently and effectively to
- perform strokes so little to no lather is left behind
- keep the nondominant thumb and fingertips dry for stretching purposes
- start strokes from a clean skin surface into the lathered surface
- wipe residual lather and hair from the razor in a safe and clean manner
- check your work for rough or missed patches

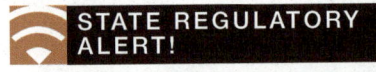

STATE REGULATORY ALERT!
Some states prohibit the use of conventional straight razors and allow only changeable-blade razors. Be guided by your state board rules and regulations.

FREEHAND POSITION AND STROKE

How to hold the razor

The position of the right hand is as follows (refer to Procedure 3):

- Take the razor in the right hand. The handle of the razor should rest between the third and fourth fingers, with the tip of the little finger resting on the tip of the tang of the razor. The thumb should sit securely on the side of the shank near the shoulder of the blade. The third finger should lie at the pivot of the shank and the handle with the first and second fingers in front of it on the back of the shank.
- Turn the hand slightly outward from the wrist with the elbow at a comfortable level.

The position of the left hand is as follows:

- Keep the fingers of the left hand dry in order to prevent them from slipping on the face.
- Use the left hand to stretch the skin in the opposite direction of the stroke under the razor.

How to perform the freehand stroke

- Use a gliding stroke toward you.
- Lead with the point of the razor in a forward, gliding movement.

Where to use the freehand stroke

- The freehand position and stroke is used in 6 of the 14 shaving areas. See Shaving Areas 1, 3, 4, 8, 11, and 12 in **Figures 12** through **17**.

BACKHAND POSITION AND STROKE

How to hold the razor

The position of the right hand is as follows:

- The shank of the razor should be held firmly between the thumb and first two fingers at the pivot with the razor held in a relatively straight position.
- The underside of the handle rests on the third and fourth fingers.
- An alternative method is to bend the handle slightly so the third finger barely rests at the end of the tang and the fourth finger is bent into the palm.
- Turn the back of the hand away from you and bend the wrist slightly downward. Then raise the elbow so that you can move the arm freely. This is the position used for the backhand stroke with the arm movement. Some practitioners prefer to use a wrist movement, in which case the arm is not held as high.

The position of the left hand is as follows:

- Keep the fingers of the left hand dry in order to prevent them from slipping.
- Stretch the skin under the razor in the opposite direction of the stroke.

How to perform the backhand stroke

- Use a gliding stroke away from you.
- Direct the stroke with the point of the razor leading in a forward, gliding movement.

Where to use the backhand stroke

The backhand stroke is used in 4 of the 14 shaving areas and if preferred, in area 12. See Shaving Areas 2, 6, 7, and 9 in **Figures 12** through **17**.

REVERSE-FREEHAND POSITION AND STROKE

The hand and razor position in the reverse-freehand stroke is similar to that of the freehand stroke, but the stroke is performed in an upward rather than a downward direction, usually with the professional standing behind the client's shoulder or head.

> **HERE'S A TIP**
> Before using the reverse-freehand stroke in Shaving Areas 5, 10, and 13, stand slightly behind the client and stroke the grain of the beard sideways to help position the hair for shaving.

How to hold the razor

The position of the right hand is as follows:

- Hold the razor firmly in a freehand position.
- Turn the hand slightly toward you so that the razor edge is turned upward

The position of the left hand is as follows:

- Keep the hand dry and use it to pull the skin taut under the razor.
- Position the fingers below or in back of the razor opposite the blade edge and direction of the stroke.

How to perform the reverse-freehand stroke

- Use an upward, semi-arced stroke toward you with the point leading in a gliding movement.
- The movement is from the elbow to the hand with a slight twist of the wrist.

Where to use the reverse-freehand stroke

The reverse-freehand stroke is used in 4 of the 14 shaving areas. See Shaving Areas 5, 10, 13, and 14 in **Figures 12** through **17**.

REVERSE-BACKHAND POSITION AND STROKE

The reverse-backhand position and stroke require diligent practice to master. The holding position of the razor for the reverse-backhand stroke is the same as that for the backhand stroke, except that the elbow is positioned downward (closer to the body) and the forearm is held upward. When using this stroke, employ a downward gliding stroke that follows along the natural hairline along the side of the neck (see **Figure 22**).

figure 22
Reverse-backhand stroke.

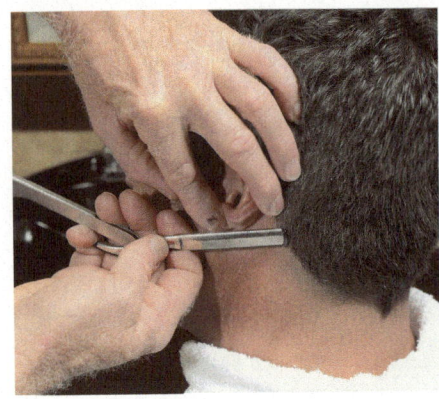

How to hold the razor

The position of the right hand is as follows:

- Hold the razor firmly in the backhand position.
- Turn the wrist to the right so that the palm of the hand faces upward.
- Drop the elbow close to the side.

The position of the left hand is as follows:

- Position the left hand so as to be able to draw the skin taut under the razor.
- Position your hand above the razor.

How to perform the reverse-backhand stroke

- Use a smooth, gliding stroke, directed downward, that leads with the point of the razor.
- Proceed with short cutting strokes directed downward and slightly outward.

Where to use the reverse-backhand stroke

The reverse-backhand stroke is only used during a neck shave with the client sitting in an upright position. Typically, the right-handed student uses a reverse-backhand stroke when shaving the client's left sideburn outline and behind the left ear along the side of the neck. The left-handed student uses a reverse-backhand stroke to shave these areas on the client's right side.

The cutting strokes described in this section illustrate the holding and stroking positions that should be employed by the right-handed student. Right-handed students start the shave on the client's right side; left-handed students start on the client's left side (see **Table 1**).

UNDERSTAND BODY POSITIONING

The shave procedure begins with the student standing at the client's side; right-handed students stand at client's right side; left-handed students stand at client's left side.

- Gently turn the client's head to the position needed to accommodate the stroke.
- Take half steps or shift your body weight from one foot to the other to change position to perform the shaving strokes; following are four common body positions with corresponding shaving areas for the right-handed student:
  - Stand slightly at front of client's right side (**Figure 23**): Shaving Areas 1, 4, and 12 (if using freehand)
  - Stand centered at client's right side (**Figure 24**): Shaving Areas 2, 3, 6, 8, 11, and 12 (if using backhand)
  - Stand at client's right shoulder (**Figure 25**): Shaving Areas 7 and 9
  - Stand behind client's right shoulder (**Figure 26**): Shaving Areas 5, 10, 13, and 14

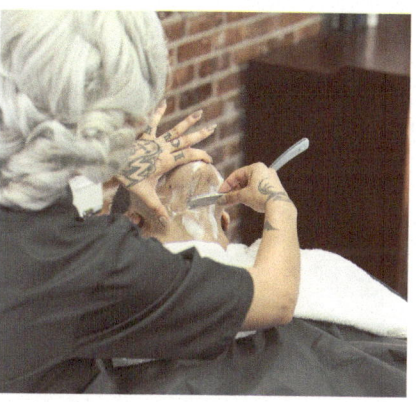
figure 23
Stand slightly at front of client's right side.

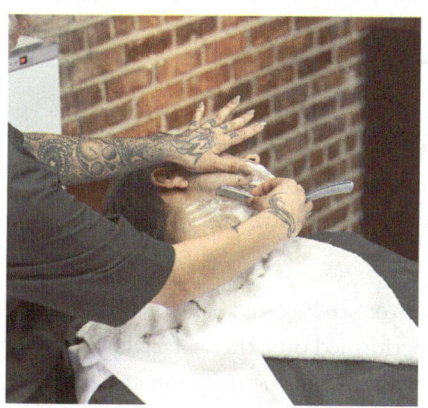
figure 24
Stand centered at client's right side.

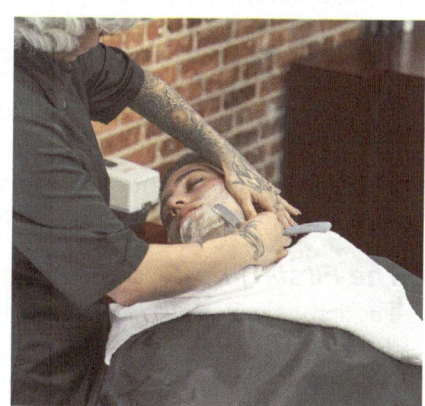
figure 25
Stand at client's right shoulder.

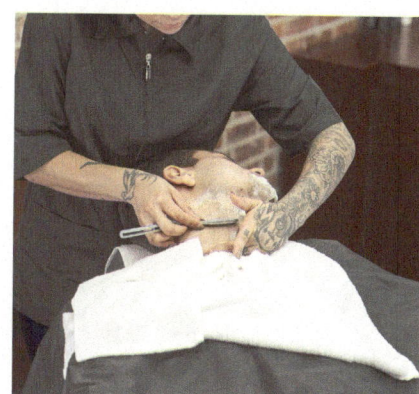
figure 26
Stand behind client's right shoulder.

DESCRIBE THE PROFESSIONAL SHAVE

The three main steps of a standard professional shave are preparation, shaving, and finishing (refer to Procedure 5). Preparation includes draping the client for the shave, preparing hot towels, and preparing the client's face for the shave.

- Draping (refer to Procedure 5: Preparation)
- Preparing hot towels
- Preparing the face for shaving involves steaming and lathering the face.
  - Steaming helps to soften the hair cuticle, provides lubrication by stimulating oil glands, and relaxes the client.
  - Lathering with a shaving cream or gel cleanses the skin, softens the hair, helps to hold the hair in an upright position for shaving, and creates a smooth surface for the razor. Use an electric latherizer to prepare warm shaving lather.

Shaving involves safely removing the hair in the 14 shaving areas without causing irritation or injury to the skin, and completing the finishing steps of the service.

- Razor strokes should be correct and systematic. Proper coordination of both hands is necessary.
- While the right hand holds and strokes the razor, the fingers of the left hand gently stretch the skin area being shaved. Taut skin allows the beard hair to be cut more easily.
- Loose skin tends to push out in front of the razor and can result in cuts or nicks. Stretching the skin too tightly, however, will cause irritation. The skin must be held firmly, neither too loosely nor too tightly, to create the correct shaving surface for the razor.
- To prevent slipping and to see the area to be shaved, remove excess lather with the thumb. If needed, dry the skin area where you will place your fingers for stretching.
- Keep the fingers of the nondominant hand dry at all times.

Finishing includes massaging moisturizer into the skin, toning to remove residual cream product, and a light powder dusting to leave a matte finish, if desired. Traditionally, a neck shave is also offered at this time.

KNOW THE TYPES OF SHAVES

There are several terms that both professionals and clients may use to describe either a type of shave or the different steps performed in a standard shave service. These terms have remained consistent for decades, so it is important that you become familiar with the terminology.

The First-Time-Over Shave

The **first-time-over shave** (FIRST-TYM-OH-ver SHAYV) is actually the primary shave in a standard shave service that is performed on lathered facial hair. The objective is to remove the beard growth without causing irritation and to leave a smooth skin surface. The *first-time-over* shave is followed by the **second-time-over shave** (SEK-und-TYM-OH-ver SHAYV) to remove any rough or uneven spots.

The Second-Time-Over Shave

The second-time-over shave is performed for one of two reasons, either as a step that follows the first-time-over shave or as part of a close shave as described in a later section (see The Close Shave). Following the first-time-over shave, check the client's skin for any rough or uneven spots. The client's skin is moistened with a warm towel or water and a freehand stroke is used to shave *with* or *across the grain* to remove any remaining hair.

The Once-Over Shave

The **once-over shave** (WONCE-OH-ver SHAYV) requires less time for a complete shave service and was popular when men patronized salons daily for their shave. This shave should result in a smooth face without being a close shave. To perform a once-over shave, use a few more strokes while shaving *across the grain* in each shaving area. This practice should ensure a complete and even shave with a single lathering. Remember to use a light hand to avoid causing irritation.

The Close Shave

Close shaving (KLOHS SHAYV-ing) is the practice of shaving the beard *against the grain* during the second-time-over phase of the shave. This practice is undesirable because it may irritate the skin and lead to infection or ingrown hairs; therefore, professionals do not traditionally employ close-shaving methods. That said, if a client's beard growth warrants it and he has requested a close shave, the professional should be able to perform the service.

The Neck Shave and the Outline Shave

A **neck shave** (NEK SHAYV) traditionally accompanies a facial shave and involves shaving the neckline on both sides of the neck behind the ears and across the nape if desired or necessary (refer to Procedure 6). Conversely, a complete *outline shave* includes the sideburn, around the ear, behind the ear areas, and sometimes the front hairline, and typically follows a haircut.

P-5 The Professional Shave *pages 34–47*

P-6 The Neck Shave *pages 48–49*

> **REMINDER**
> Be sure to check the hairline and neck areas for moles, warts, or other hypertrophies before beginning the neck shave; follow the natural hairline for best results.

Understand Facial-Hair Design

LO 10 Describe the differences between various facial-hair designs.

In addition to cutting and styling hair, you should be able to offer your clients a full range of services for grooming facial hair. Because today's style is one of individuality, students should become proficient, or even specialize, in the design and trimming of men's facial hair. The client who wears a mustache and/or beard will frequent a shop that can provide both haircutting and facial-hair design services.

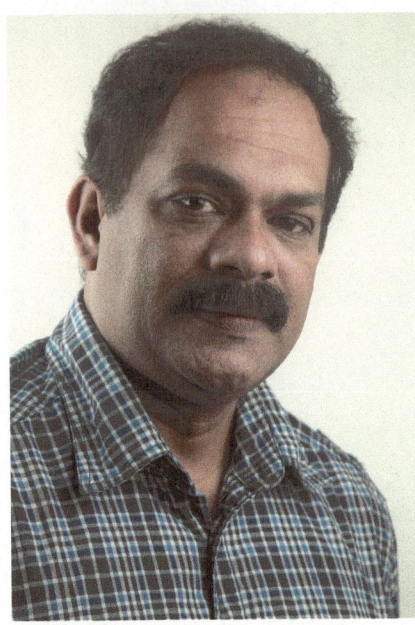

figure 27
Thicker mustache design for heavier facial features.

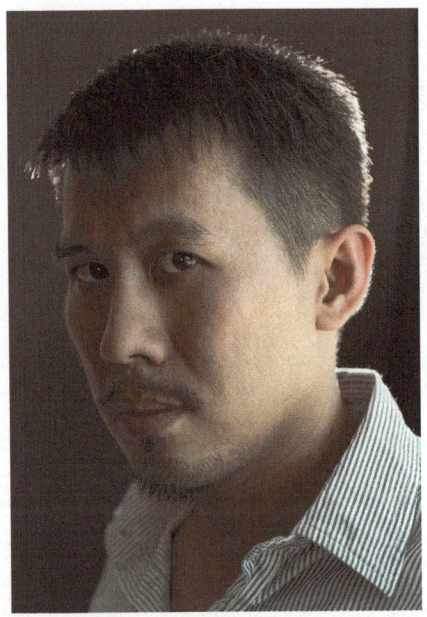

figure 28
Thinner mustache design for finer facial features.

TRIMMING THE MUSTACHE

A mustache is most often worn for personal adornment and men are usually very particular about how it is designed and maintained. Care, artistry, and sensitivity to the client's preferences are required for this service. Corrective shaping or redesign of the mustache can help clients with their daily maintenance and trimming until their next visit to the salon.

In addition to knowing how to trim and shape mustaches, professionals should be able to understand and apply certain principles of mustache design.

Mustache Design

Factors to consider when consulting with a client about suitable mustache designs are his facial features, hair growth and texture, and personal taste. Consider the following factors when discussing mustache design options with your client:

- The size of the mustache should correspond to the size of the client's features, for example, larger, thicker designs for heavier facial features and smaller, thinner designs for finer features (Figures 27 and 28).
- Following are important facial characteristics that influence mustache design:
  - Width of the mouth
  - Size of the nose
  - Shape of upper lip area
  - Width of the cheeks, jaw, and chin
  - Density and texture of hair growth
- As a general rule, be guided by the client's hair growth pattern and avoid cutting too deeply into natural hairlines. This approach will help to minimize daily maintenance as new growth occurs.
- Following are guidelines for mustache design and proportion:
  - *Large, coarse facial features:* heavier-looking mustache
  - *Prominent nose:* medium to large mustache
  - *Long, narrow face:* narrow to medium mustache
  - *Extra-large mouth:* pyramid-shaped mustache
  - *Extra-small mouth:* medium, short mustache
  - *Smallish, regular features:* smaller, triangular mustache
  - *Wide mouth with prominent upper lip:* heavier handlebar or large divided mustache
  - *Round face with regular features:* semisquare mustache
  - *Square with prominent features:* heavier, linear mustache with ends slightly curving downward
- Additional services that may be offered with a mustache trim include:
  - waxing mustache ends;
  - penciling with temporary color;
  - coloring for evenness or compatibility with scalp hair color.

DESIGNING THE BEARD

Like mustaches, beards can be used to balance the appearance of facial features. As with their mustaches, men are usually very particular about the design of their beards. Again, a careful approach, artistry, and sensitivity to the client's preferences are required for this service.

If the client is getting a haircut along with his beard trim, the decision must be made as to which service will be performed first. This is completely a matter of choice; you will have your own reasons for performing one service before or after the other. For example, many professionals cut and style the hair before the beard trim so they can balance the length and fullness of the beard with the finished haircut more effectively.

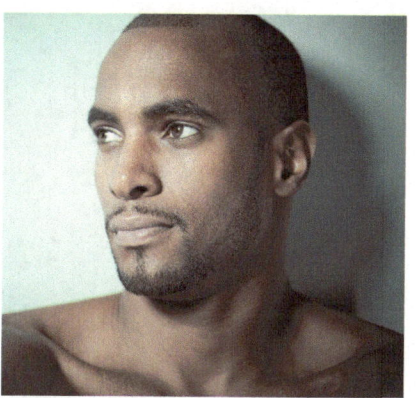

figure 29
A balanced and proportioned beard design.

Beard Design

The correct shaping or design of the beard can emphasize pleasant facial features, minimize less desirable ones, and camouflage flaws. As with other hair design, it is important to develop a good eye for balance and proportion (**Figure 29**). Since very few individuals have perfectly symmetrical face shapes, it may be challenging to create the illusion of symmetry and balance in design. Following are some important practical tips for beard design:

- Analyze the density and distribution of the hair to identify uneven growth areas; cutting the hair too short in the area surrounding these sections will result in emphasizing the *bald spot* with no way to provide coverage of the uneven area.

- Work with the natural hairline in the sideburn, cheek, and mustache areas to guide the design and to minimize daily maintenance.

- Consider where hair growth under the chin and jaw changes direction to help determine design options for outlines in this area.

- Leave the facial hair slightly longer than the desired end result during the first trimming to avoid cutting the hair too closely. Remember, you can always cut more off. This is also a good time to face the client to the mirror so he can check the progress of the trim and to clarify or ask anything you need to know to finish the service.

- Beard trimming and design is usually performed with a combination of the shears, comb, outliner and/or clippers, and razor.

- Even-all-over clipper-cutting is most successful on beards with even density and texture. This is important to note because sometimes cutting the beard at all the same length will leave whorls or patches, especially in wavy hair.

  - When creating a uniform length throughout the beard, start with a blade size close to the length of the client's beard. If more than a light trim is required, select the next size blade that will cut the hair to a shorter length. Repeat as necessary until the desired length is achieved.

  - Follow up clipper work with shears, outliner, and/or razor for final trimming and detail work.

Perfecting your mustache and beard design skills will help you meet the service needs of your clients while providing an outlet for creative design and an additional income source (refer to Procedures 7 and 8).

> **? DID YOU KNOW?**
> **Styptic powder** (STIP-tik POW-dur) or liquid, made from alum, is an antihemorrhagic with astringent properties that can stop the bleeding of small nicks or cuts.

figure 30
Head shaving has grown in popularity.

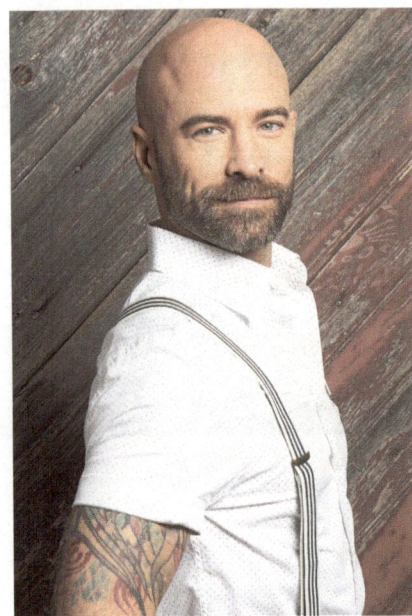

-7 **Mustache Trim** page 50

-8 **Beard Designs** pages 51–56

DISCUSS HEAD SHAVING

The shaved head is one of today's fashion trends that many men choose regardless of the density or growth pattern of their hair (**Figure 30**). The hair and scalp are prepared with hot towels and lather followed by straight-razor shaving. Following are some guidelines for performing a head shave:

- Thoroughly analyze the scalp to identify moles and other hypertrophies.
- If you are precutting the hair, leave enough length for the razor to grab as the blade passes over the scalp.
- Keep the scalp moist and your stretching (nondominant) hand dry.
- Stretch the skin to create a smooth shaving surface.

-9 **Arching Technique with Razor** pages 57–58

-10 **Outline Shave** pages 59–61

-11 **The Head Shave** pages 62–65

Review Shaving-Related Infection Control and Safety Precautions

After reading the next section, you will be able to:

LO 11 Discuss infection control and safety precautions associated with shaving.

Use **Table 2** as a guide for complying with infection control and safety precautions associated with shaving as you perform the procedures.

24 MILADY STANDARD SHAVING

table 2
INFECTION CONTROL AND SAFETY PRECAUTIONS

- Clean and disinfect razors and blades before use.
- Discard used blades in a sharps container.
- Wash your hands before servicing a client.
- Use clean linens, capes, and paper products.
- Provide a clean cloth or paper barrier between the client's head and the headrest.
- Treat small cuts or nicks using standard precautions and exposure incident procedures.
- Lock the chair once the client is properly draped and in position for the shave.
- Prepare facial hair for the shave with warm or hot towels and lather.
- Use a light touch and a forward gliding motion that leads with the point of the blade.
- Observe the hair growth pattern and shave with it, not against it.
- Lather against the grain *gently* to place the hair in a position to be shaved.
- Keep your fingers dry to stretch or hold the skin firmly during the shave.
- Use the cushions of the fingertips to stretch skin in the opposite direction of the razor stroke.
- Keep the fingers and thumb of the nondominant hand away from the path of the razor.
- Apply lather neatly to the areas to be shaved and replace as necessary.
- Keep the skin moist while shaving.
- Follow through with shaving strokes from one shaving area to another; do not stop short or shave over an area repeatedly.

AN EXPOSURE INCIDENT: CONTACT WITH BLOOD OR BODY FLUID

You should never perform a service on any client who comes into the shop with an open wound, a rash, or an abrasion. Sometimes accidents happen while a service is being performed in the salon, however.

An **exposure incident** (eks-POH-zhoor in-SI-dent) is contact with non-intact (broken) skin, blood, body fluid, or other potentially infectious materials that is the result of the performance of a worker's duties. Should the client suffer a cut or abrasion that bleeds during a service, follow the steps outlined in Procedure 12 for the client's safety, as well as your own.

P-12 **Handling an Exposure Incident** *pages 66*

HONING THE RAZOR

MATERIALS, IMPLEMENTS, AND EQUIPMENT

- ☐ Conventional straight razor
- ☐ Hone
- ☐ Shaving lather
- ☐ Water

PROCEDURE

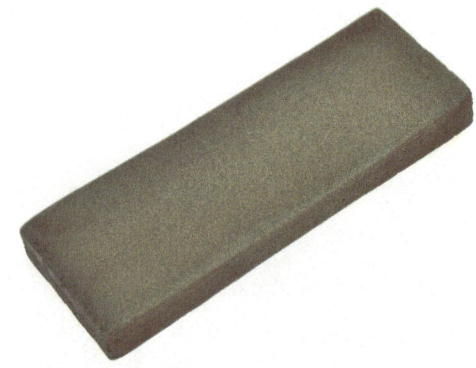

1. Position the hone by placing it firmly and flatly on a hard, smooth surface.

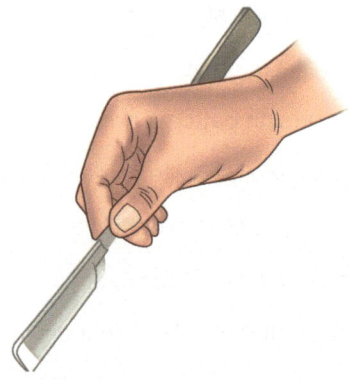

2. Grasp the razor handle comfortably in your dominant hand as follows:
   a. Rest the index finger on top of the side part of the shank.
   b. Rest the ball of the thumb at the joint.
   c. Place the second finger at the back of the razor near the edge of the shank.
   d. Fold the remaining fingers around the handle to permit easy turning of the razor.

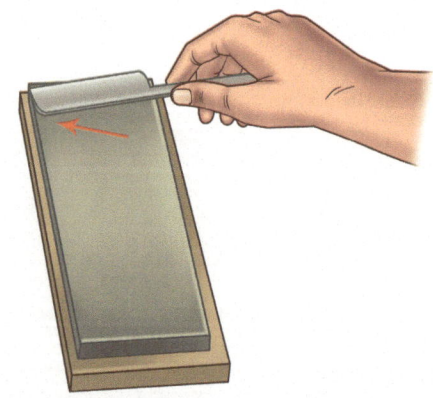

3. *First position and stroke:* Place the razor on its back on the upper far left corner of the hone.

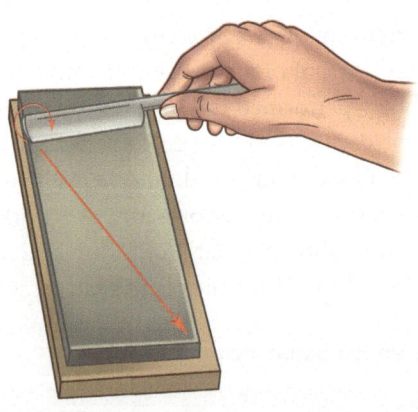

4. Roll the razor, using the thumb and index finger to position the blade edge flat against the hone and facing toward you. Draw the blade diagonally across the hone from heel to point.

PROCEDURE 1

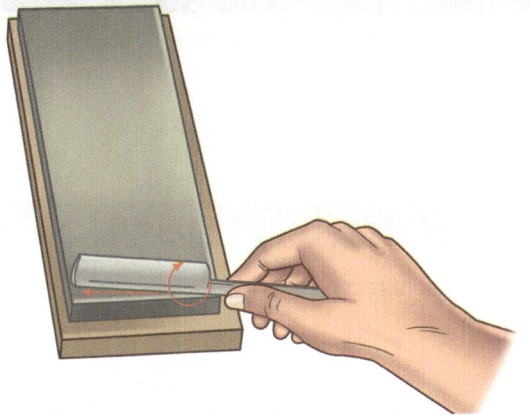

5 Turn the razor on its back and slide it toward the bottom left corner of the hone to position it for the second position and stroke.

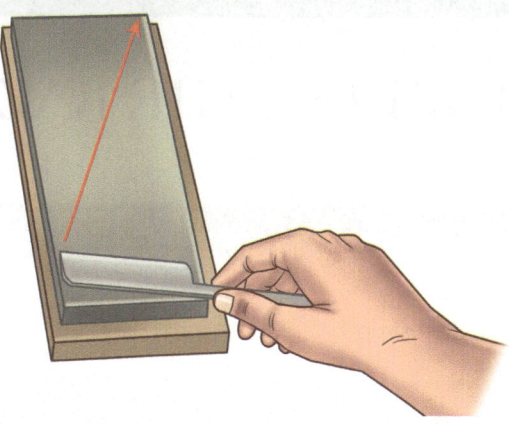

6 *Second position and stroke:* Begin at lower left corner of the hone with the blade edge flat against the hone and facing away from you.

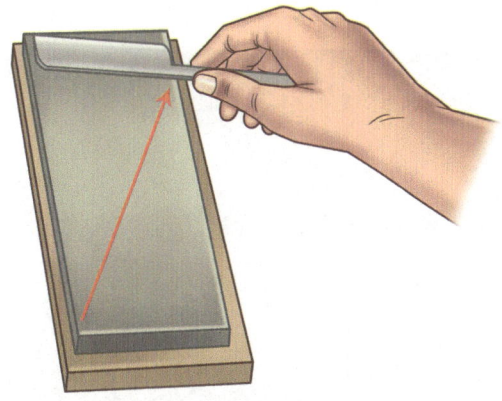

7 Stroke the blade diagonally toward the upper right corner of the hone.

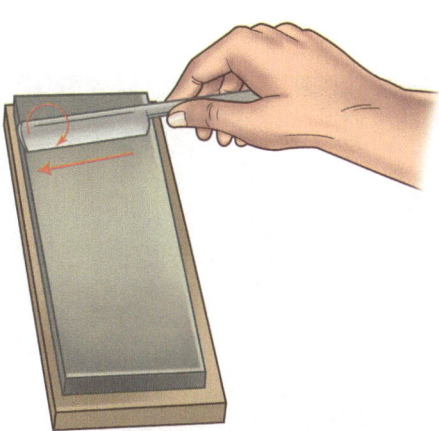

8 Turn the razor on its back, slide it toward the upper left corner of the hone, and roll it into position for the next stroke.

9 Repeat the strokes in a slow and rhythmic manner with equal pressure. If the razor is very dull, use firm pressure during the first honing strokes and then decrease the pressure as the razor takes an edge.

10 Test the edge by lightly passing it over a thumbnail moistened with water or lather.

STROPPING THE RAZOR

MATERIALS, IMPLEMENTS, AND EQUIPMENT

- ☐ Barber chair
- ☐ Combination strop
- ☐ Conventional straight razor

PROCEDURE

1 Clip the strop onto the arm of the chair. Hold the end of the strop firmly in the left hand on a slight diagonal from the chair and as high as is comfortable.

2 Grasp the razor firmly in the right hand with the thumb and index finger at the shank and the handle in your palm.

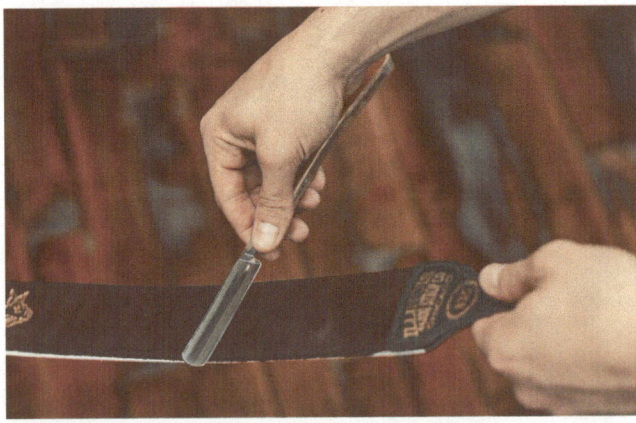

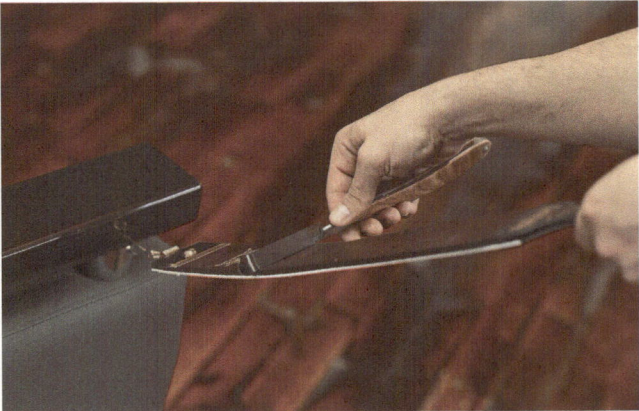

3 *First stroke:* Start the stroke at the top edge of the strop closest to the hand. Using a long, diagonal stroke with even pressure from the heel to the point, draw the razor perfectly flat, with back leading, straight over the surface. Bear down just heavily enough to feel the razor draw.

4 *Second stroke:* When the first stroke is completed, turn the razor on the back of the blade by rolling it between the fingers without turning the hand.

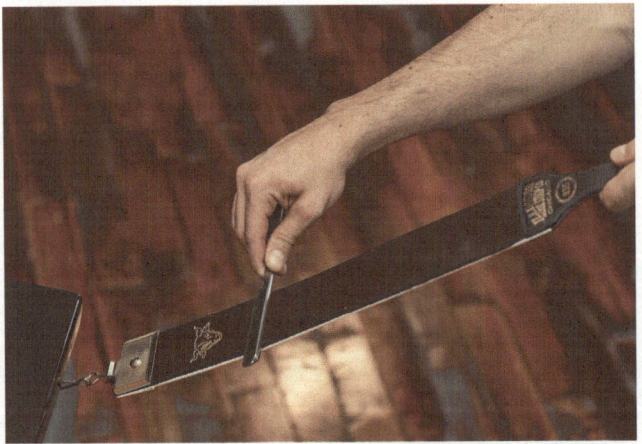

5 Draw the razor away from the chair toward you to complete the second stroke. Repeat strokes as necessary.

6 Make a final test of the razor prior to shaving on the moistened tip of the thumb.

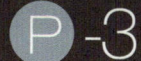

HANDLING A STRAIGHT RAZOR

After practicing this procedure, you should be able to:

LO 12 Demonstrate how to handle a straight razor safely.

Note: The first step in learning how to shave is to master the fundamentals of handling the razor. Review the parts of the razor to become familiar with terms associated with this tool.

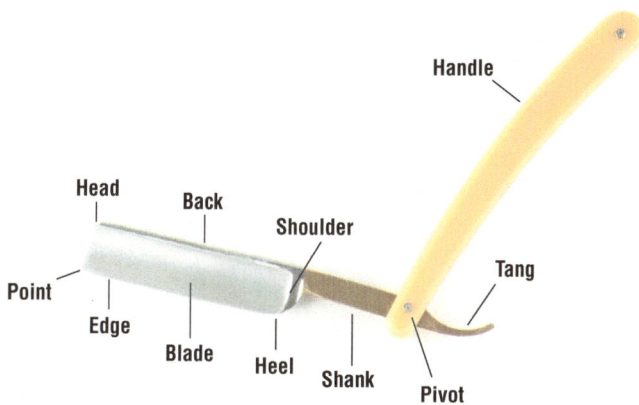

MATERIALS, IMPLEMENTS, AND EQUIPMENT	PREPARATION
☐ Straight razor with blade	1. Assemble supplies.
	2. Wash your hands.

PROCEDURE

1. To open the razor, grasp the back of the blade between the thumb and index finger of the dominant hand while holding the handle with the opposite thumb and index finger.

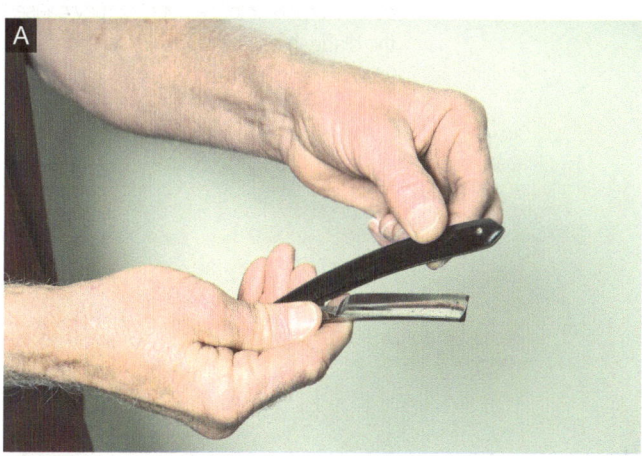

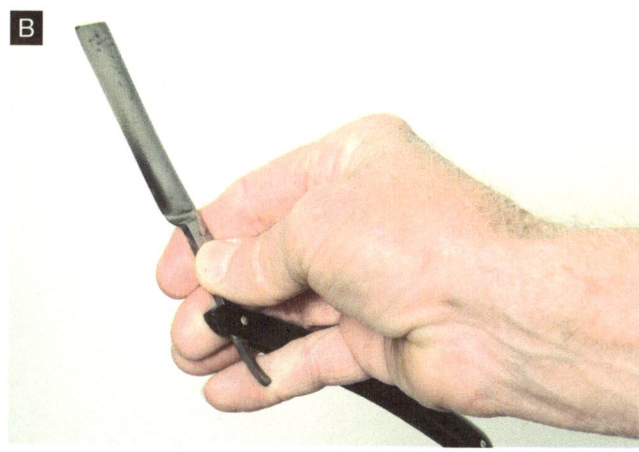

2. As the blade and handle separate by way of the pivot, reposition the little finger of the dominant hand to rest on the tang as the handle is placed in an upward position.

PROCEDURE 3

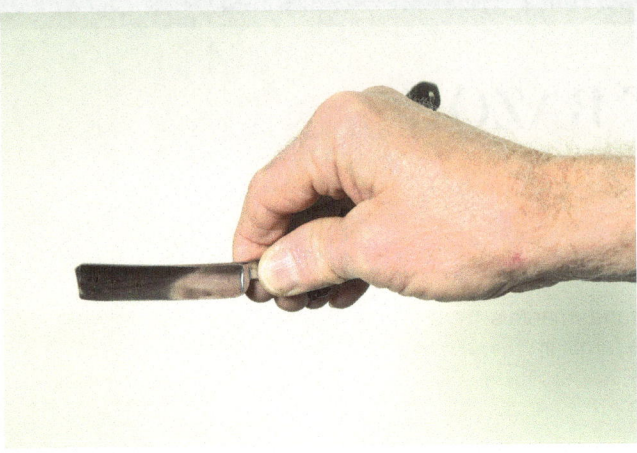

③ Hold the razor between the thumb and index finger on the sides of the shank near the shoulder of the blade and rest across the second and third fingers, with the little finger bracing the razor.

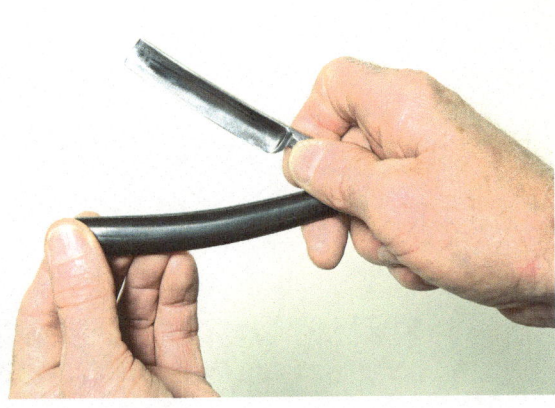

④ When closing the razor, release the little finger and bring the handle to the blade. Be careful the cutting edge does not strike the handle.

CLEAN-UP AND DISINFECTION

- ☐ Clean and disinfect the tools and implements.
- ☐ Clean and then disinfect the work area.
- ☐ Deposit used blades in a sharps container.
- ☐ Dispose of single-use items. Place all used linens, towels, and capes in the laundry.
- ☐ Wash your hands.

> ⚠ **CAUTION**
> Always handle razors with extreme care. Warped or loose handles may cause the blade to pass through to the fingers when closing the razor.

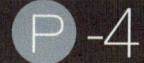 P-4

RAZOR POSITION AND STROKES PRACTICE

After practicing this procedure, you should be able to:

LO 13 Demonstrate the freehand, backhand, reverse-freehand, and reverse-backhand positions and strokes.

Note: After mastering this procedure, repeat the steps using a bladed straight razor on a live model (or as directed by your instructor) before advancing to Procedure 5.

MATERIALS, IMPLEMENTS, AND EQUIPMENT

☐ Beardless male mannequin and stand ☐ Straight razor (without a blade)

PREPARATION

① Assemble supplies. ② Wash your hands.

PROCEDURE

A. FREEHAND POSITION AND STROKE

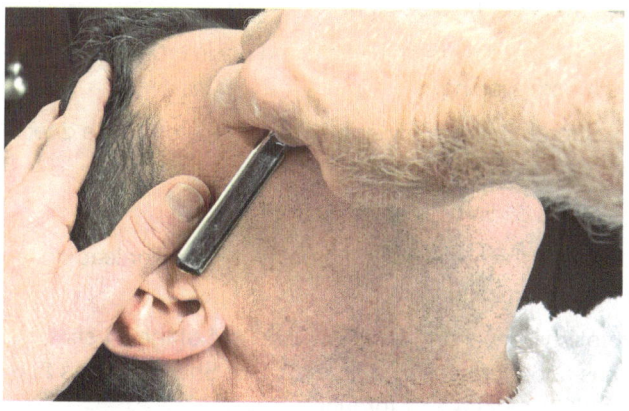

① Hold the razor in the right hand. The handle should rest between the third and fourth fingers, with the tip of the little finger resting on the tip of the tang. The thumb should sit securely on the side of the shank near the shoulder of the blade. The third finger should lie at the pivot with the first and second fingers in front of it on the back of the shank.

② Turn the hand slightly outward from the wrist with the elbow at a comfortable level.

③ Keep the fingers of the left hand dry to prevent slipping.

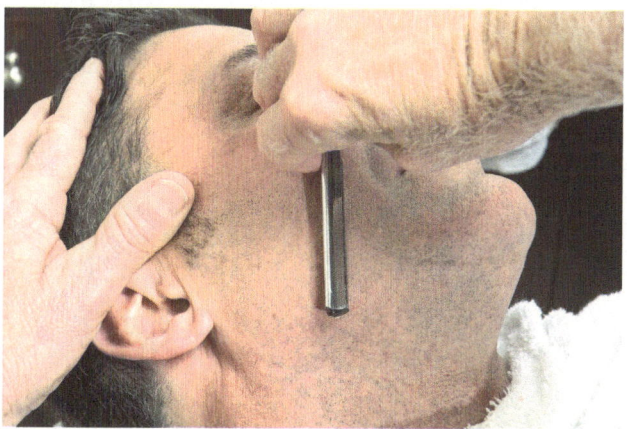

④ Use the left hand to stretch the skin in the opposite direction of the stroke.

⑤ Use a gliding stroke toward you.

⑥ Lead with the point of the razor in a forward, gliding movement.

Note: The freehand position and stroke is used in 6 of the 14 shaving areas. See Shaving Areas 1, 3, 4, 8, 11, and 12 in Figures 12 through 17.

B. BACKHAND POSITION AND STROKE

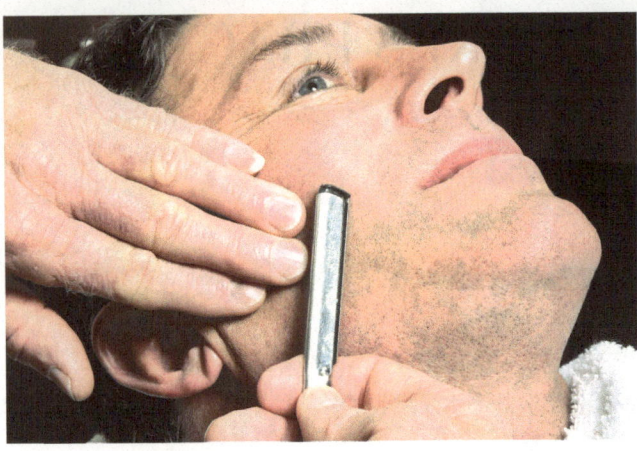

7 The shank of the razor should be held firmly between the thumb and first two fingers at the pivot with the razor held in a relatively straight position.

8 The underside of the handle rests on the third and fourth fingers.

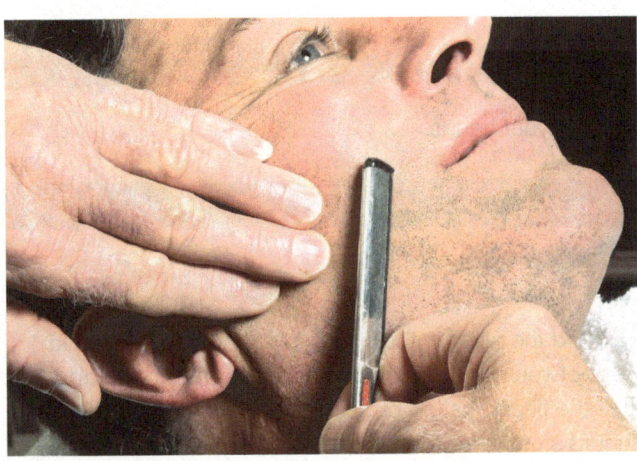

9 An alternative method is to bend the handle slightly so the third finger barely rests at the end of the tang and the fourth finger is bent into the palm.

10 Turn the back of the hand away from you and bend the wrist slightly downward. Then raise the elbow so that you can move the arm freely. This is the position used for the backhand stroke with the arm movement. Some practitioners prefer to use a wrist movement, in which case the arm is not held as high.

11 Keep the fingers of the left hand dry in order to prevent them from slipping.

12 Stretch the skin under the razor in the opposite direction of the stroke.

13 Use a gliding stroke away from you.

14 Direct the stroke with the point of the razor leading in a forward, gliding movement.

Note: The backhand stroke is used in 4 of the 14 shaving areas and if preferred, in area 12. See Shaving Areas 2, 6, 7, and 9 in Figures 12 through 17.

C. REVERSE-FREEHAND POSITION AND STROKE

The hand and razor position of the reverse-freehand stroke is similar to that of the freehand stroke, but the stroke is performed in an upward rather than a downward direction, usually with the professional standing at the client's shoulder or behind the client's head.

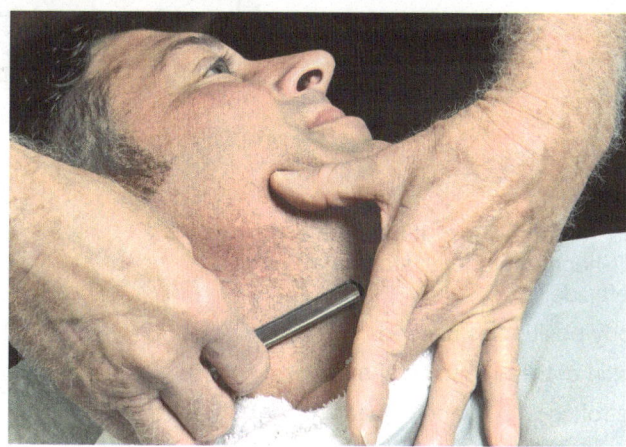

15 Hold the razor firmly in a freehand position.

16 Turn the hand slightly toward you so that the razor edge is turned upward.

17 Keep the hand dry and use it to pull the skin taut under the razor.

18 Position the fingers below or at the back of the razor opposite to the blade edge and direction of the stroke.

19 Use an upward, semi-arced stroke toward you in a gliding movement.

20 The movement is from the elbow to the hand with a slight twist of the wrist.

Note: The reverse-freehand stroke is used in 4 of the 14 shaving areas. See Shaving Areas 5, 10, 13, and 14 in Figures 12 through 17.

D. REVERSE-BACKHAND POSITION AND STROKE

The holding position of the razor for the reverse-backhand stroke is the same as the backhand stroke except that the elbow is positioned downward (closer to the body) and the forearm in held upward. When using this stroke, employ a downward gliding stroke that follows along the natural hairline along the side of the neck.

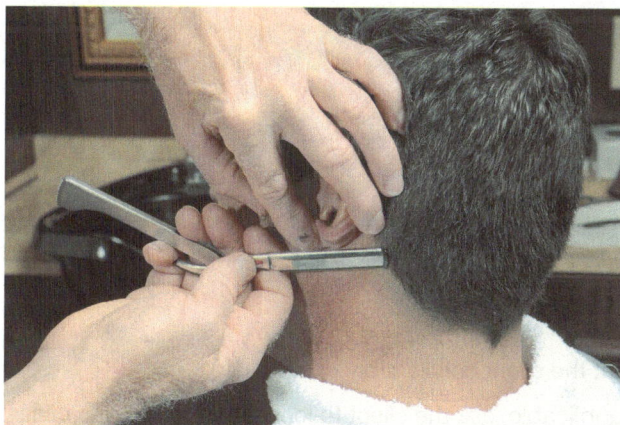

21 Hold the razor firmly in the backhand position.

22 Turn the wrist so that the palm faces upward.

23 Drop the elbow close to the side.

24 Position the left hand so as to be able to draw the skin taut under the razor.

25 Position your hand above the razor.

26 Use a smooth, gliding stroke.

27 Direct the stroke downward along the side of the neck.

Note: The reverse-backhand stroke is used for shaving the left side behind the ear along the side of the neck by the right-handed person and on the right side along the side of the neck by the left-handed person.

CLEAN-UP AND DISINFECTION

- ☐ Clean and disinfect the tools and implements.
- ☐ Clean and then disinfect the work area.
- ☐ Deposit used blades in a sharps container.
- ☐ Dispose of single-use items. Place all used linens, towels, and capes in the laundry.
- ☐ Wash your hands.

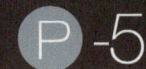

THE PROFESSIONAL SHAVE

After practicing this procedure, you should be able to:

LO14 Demonstrate a shave service.

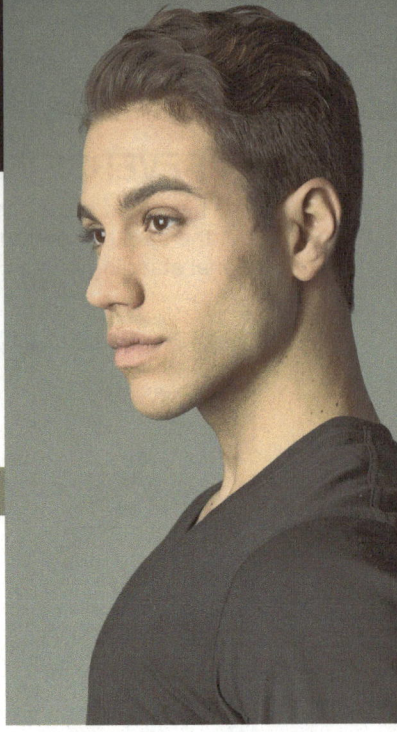

REMINDERS

- Analyze the client's skin and hair growth patterns.
- Keep client's skin moist.
- Keep your fingers dry.
- Position the client's head as needed.
- Remove excess lather with thumb before beginning stroke.
- Right-handed students stand at the client's right side; left-handed students stand at the client's left side.
- Shift your body position as needed.
- Stretch the skin of the area to be shaved.
- Use gliding strokes with the point leading.

MATERIALS, IMPLEMENTS, AND EQUIPMENT

- Barber chair with headrest
- Comb and brush
- Cotton pledgets or tissues
- Covered container for soiled towels
- Covered trash can
- Electric latherizer
- Haircutting cape
- Headrest cover
- Hot-towel cabinet
- Moisturizing cream
- Paper towels
- Sharps container
- Shaving cream or gel
- Sink
- Straight razor and blades
- Terry cloth towels
- Toner or astringent

PREPARATION

1. Assemble supplies.
2. Wash your hands.

PROCEDURE

A. PREPARE CLIENT FOR THE SHAVE

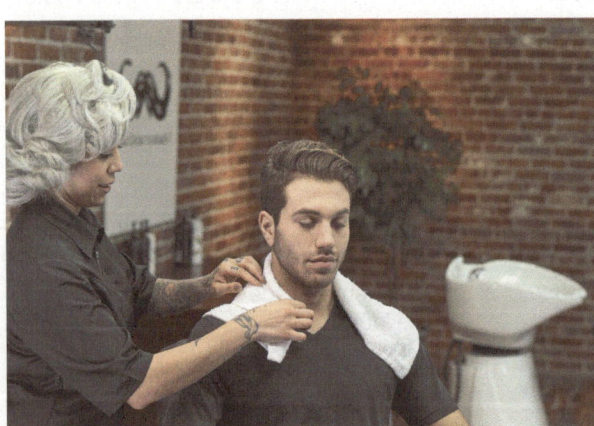

1. Seat the client comfortably in the chair.
2. If applicable, ask the client to loosen his collar; turn collar to inside. Position a terry cloth towel from back to front.

34   MILADY STANDARD SHAVING

PROCEDURE 5

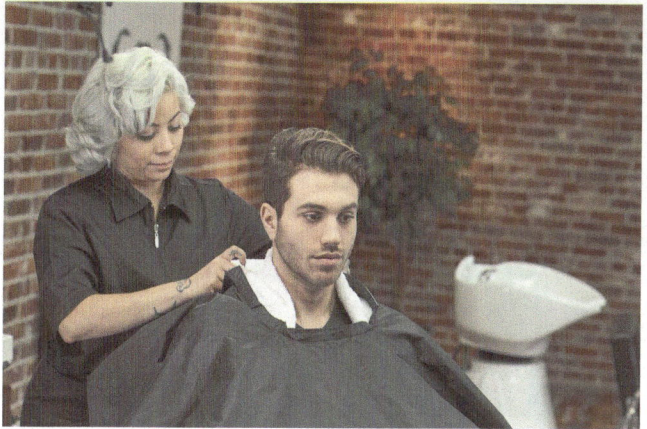

3 Lay the cape loosely over the client's shoulders from the front without it coming into contact with the client's neck.

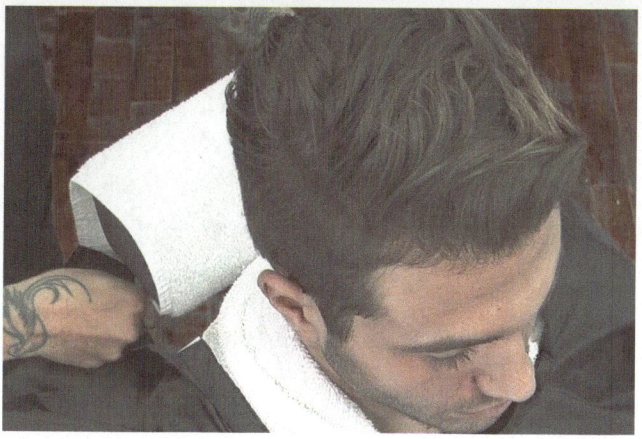

4 Apply a fresh headrest cover and adjust the headrest to the proper height.

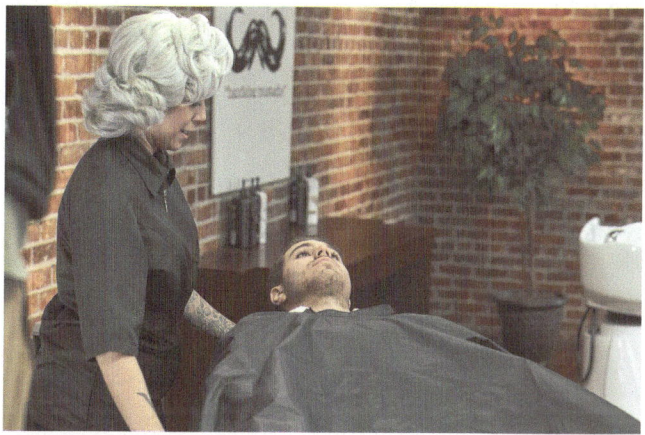

5 Recline the chair to a comfortable working angle for you and the client.

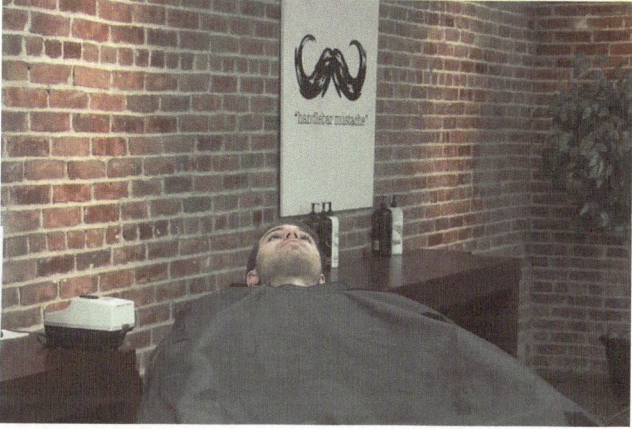

6 Adjust and lock the chair to the proper height.

7 Wash your hands with soap and warm water, and dry them thoroughly.

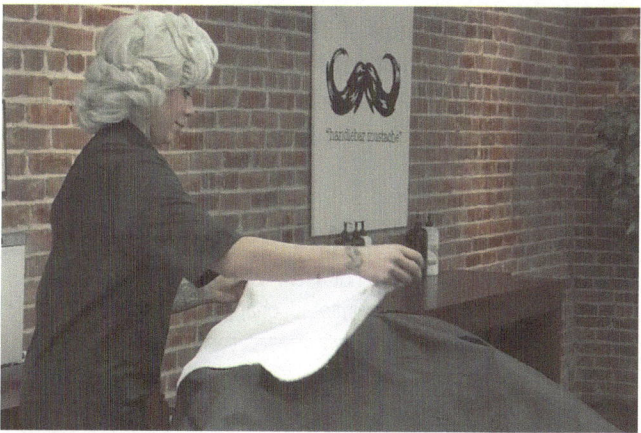

8 Unfold a clean terry cloth towel, and lay it diagonally across the client's chest.

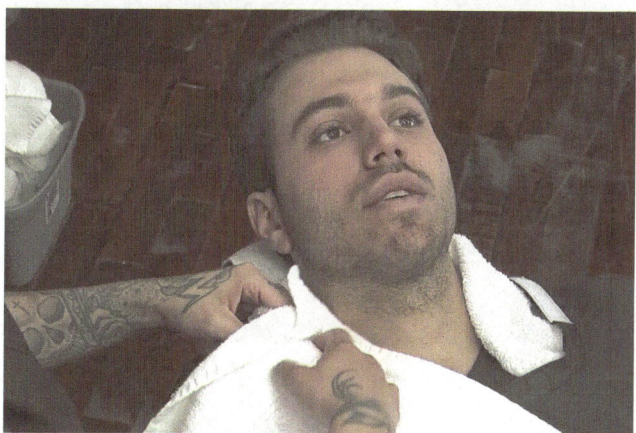

9 Tuck one corner of the towel along the right side of the client's neck. Secure the tucked edge by sliding a finger inside the neckband.

MILADY STANDARD SHAVING

PROCEDURE 5

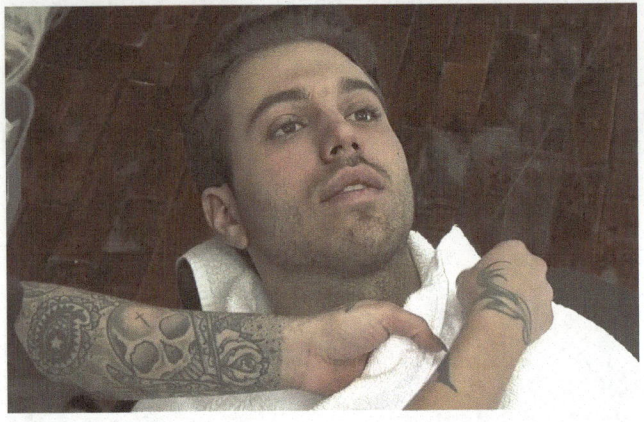

10 Cross the lower end of the towel to the other side of the client's neck and tuck under the neckband using the same sliding motion.

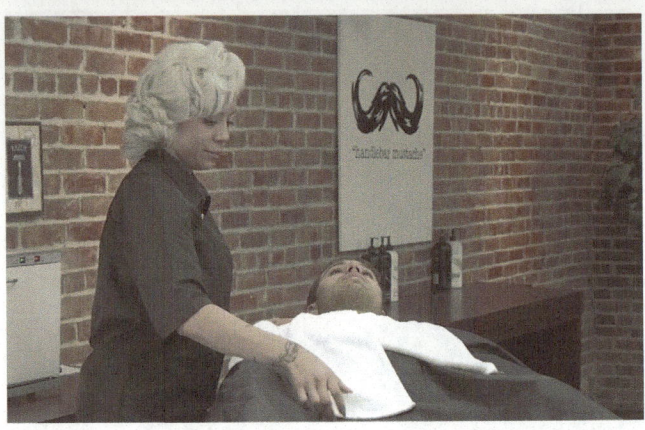

11 Tuck a paper strip or paper towel into the neckband and lay it across the client's chest. Use for wiping the razor clean during the shave.

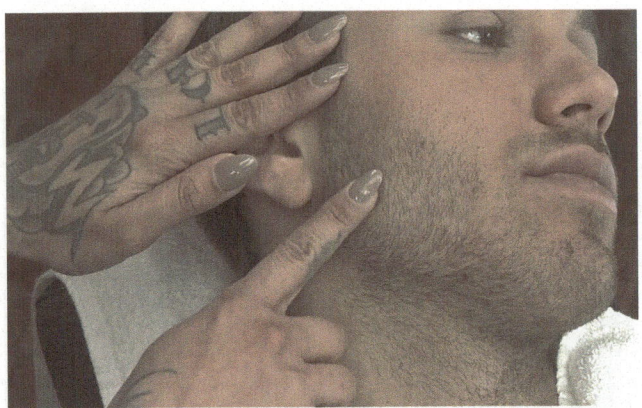

12 Analyze client's skin, hair texture, and hair growth patterns.

B. PREPARE CLIENT'S FACE FOR SHAVING

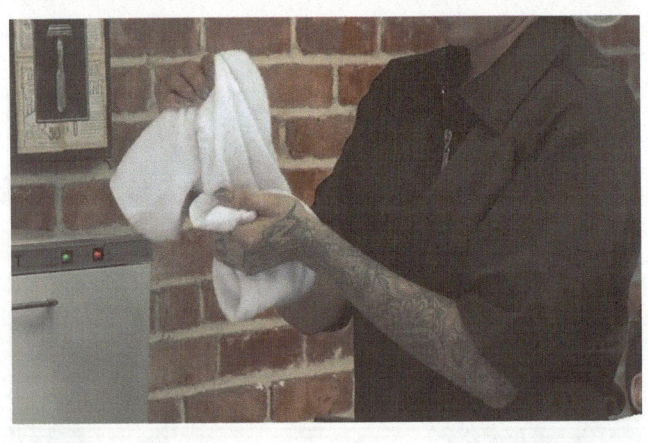

13 Retrieve a pre-warmed towel from the hot-towel cabinet.

14 Test the temperature of the towel on your wrist. If it is too hot, hold the towel by the top corners and gently fan it back and forth for a few seconds. Test the towel again before applying it to the client's face.

> ⚠ **CAUTION**
> Do not use a hot steam towel if the skin is sensitive, irritated, chapped, or blistered.

PROCEDURE 5

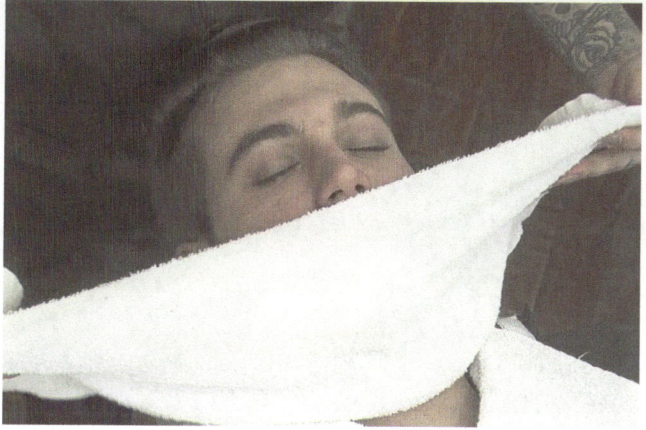

15 Standing behind the client's head, position the hot towel under and in front of the client's chin. Fold the towel over the client's mouth and upper lip area to just under his nose.

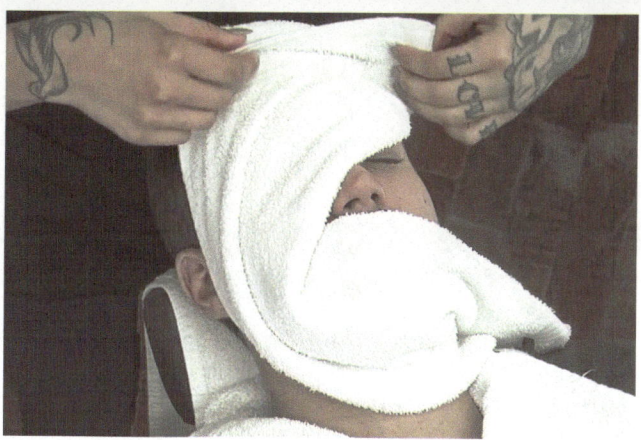

16 Cross the right-hand section of the towel over to the client's right temple area.

A

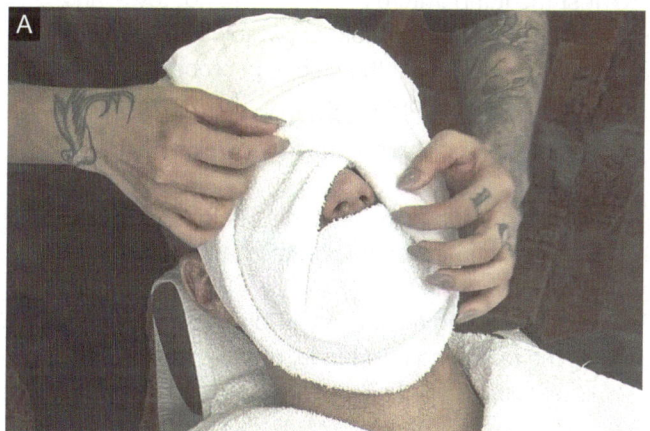

B

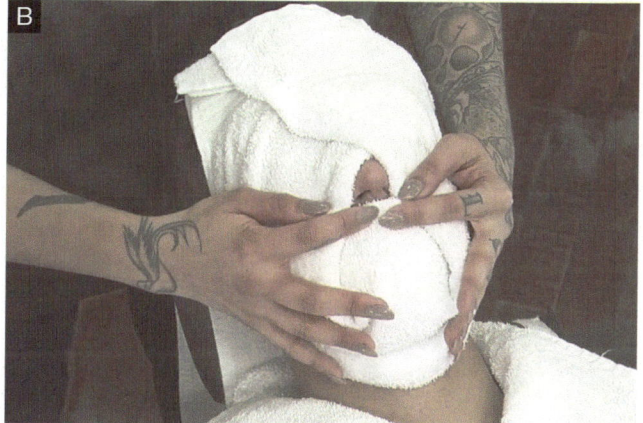

17 Bring the left-hand section of the towel over toward the client's left side and smooth the fold. Mold towel to client's face.

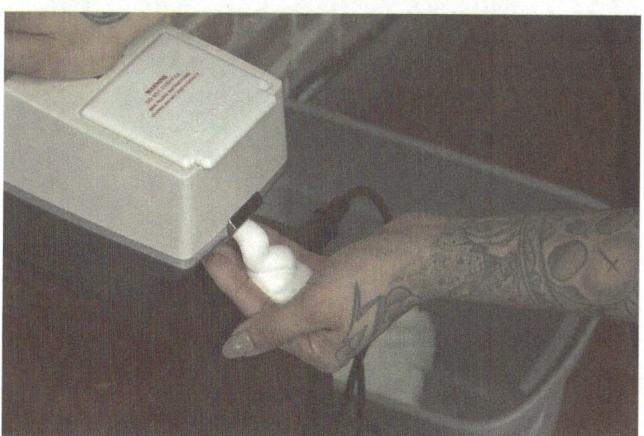

18 Transfer a quantity of warm shaving lather from the electric latherizer into your hand.

19 Remove the hot towel, and spread lather evenly over the bearded areas to be shaved.

MILADY STANDARD SHAVING

PROCEDURE 5

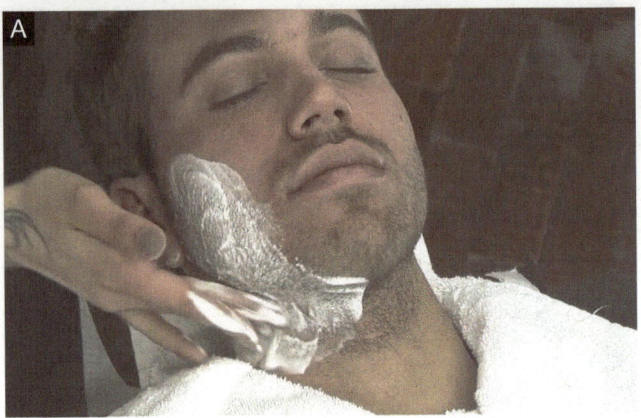
A

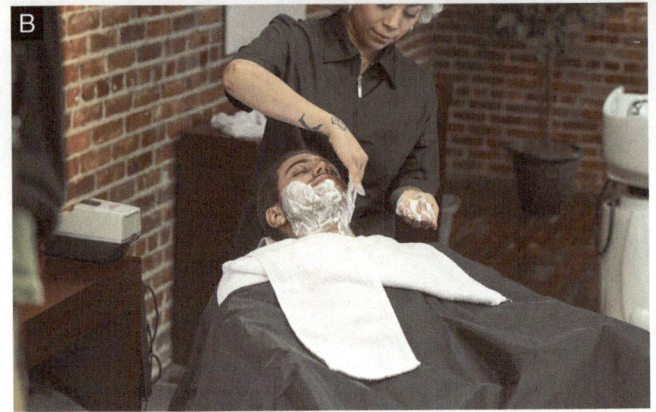
B

20 Starting at the neck and working up the right side of the face, use brisk, rotary movements with the cushions of the fingertips to work the shaving cream into a lather in the bearded areas of the face. Repeat on the left side of the neck and face until all areas to be shaved are covered. Rub for 1 to 2 minutes depending on the stiffness and density of the beard.

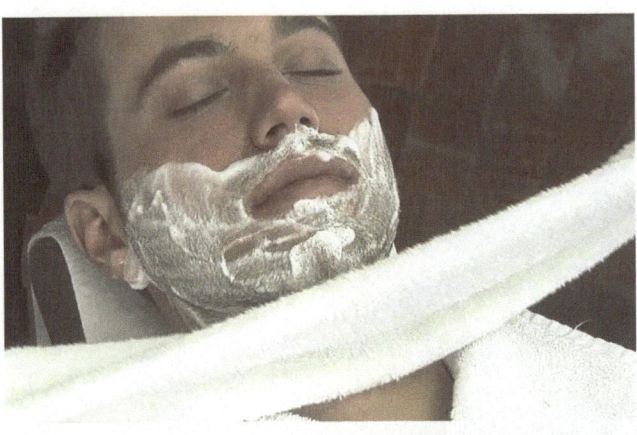

21 Test the temperature of the second hot towel and apply it over the lather. Mold or pat towel to conform to client's face. Repeat the steaming process if the beard is extremely coarse or dense.

22 Prepare the razor while the hot towel is on the client's face.
   a. When using a conventional straight razor, strop the razor, immerse it in a disinfectant solution, rinse, and wipe dry.
   b. When using a changeable-blade razor, disinfect the razor and new blade, rinse, wipe dry, and assemble.

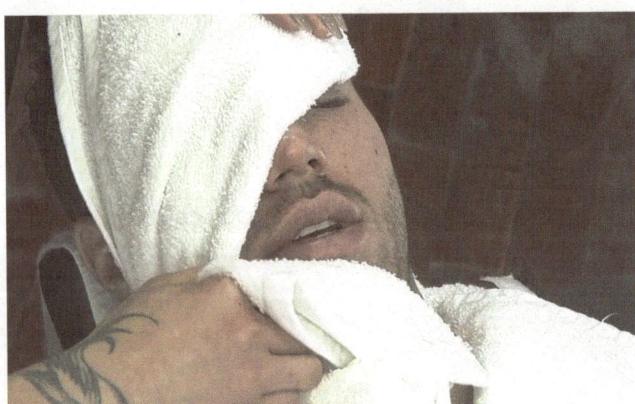

23 Remove hot towel and wipe the lather off in one smooth operation.

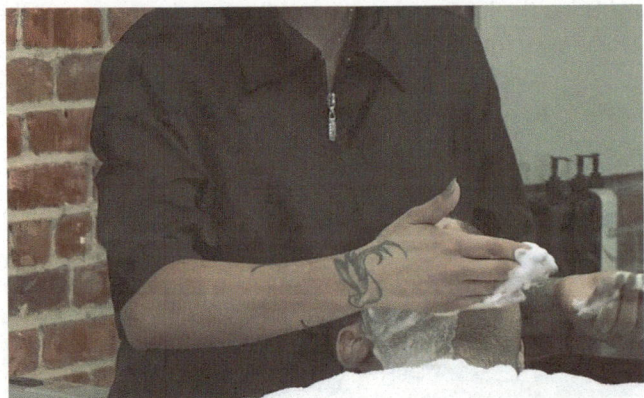

24 Re-lather the beard and wipe the lather from your hands.

38　MILADY STANDARD SHAVING

C. THE FACIAL SHAVE

First-Time-Over Shave

Shaving Area No. 1—Freehand stroke

> **CAUTION**
> Avoid sawing, scraping, pushing, or sideways movements with straight razors to avoid causing injury to the skin. Always employ a gentle gliding motion that leads with the point of the blade.

25 Stand at the right side of chair and shift weight to right foot; gently turn the client's face to the left. Remove the lather from the hairline with the thumb of the left hand. Hold the razor in a freehand position.

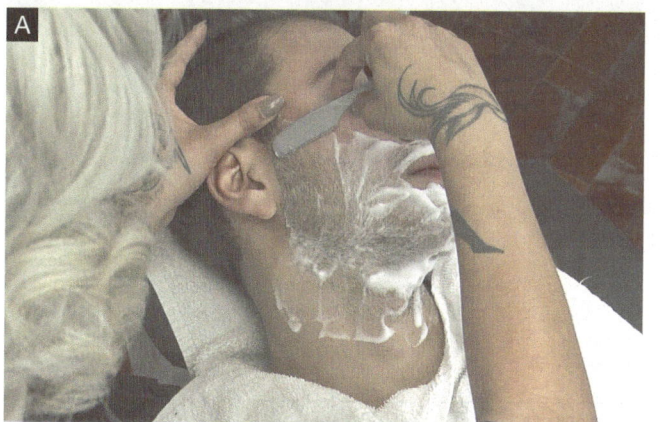
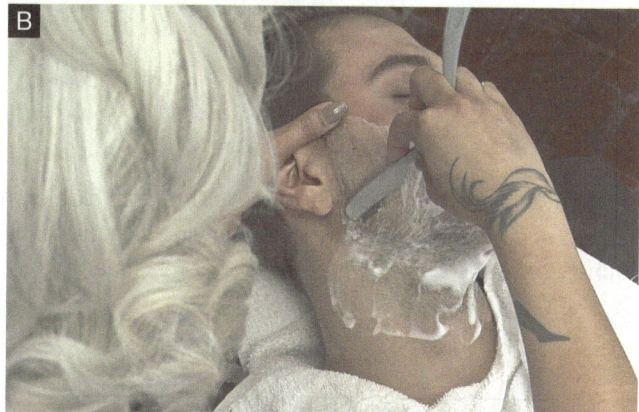

26 Stretch the skin and begin at the hairline of the right sideburn. Use a gliding diagonal stroke that leads with the point of the razor; shave downward toward the corner of the mouth and jawbone.

27 Wipe razor clean.

Shaving Area No. 2—Backhand stroke

28 Shift your weight to the left foot; hold razor in backhand position.

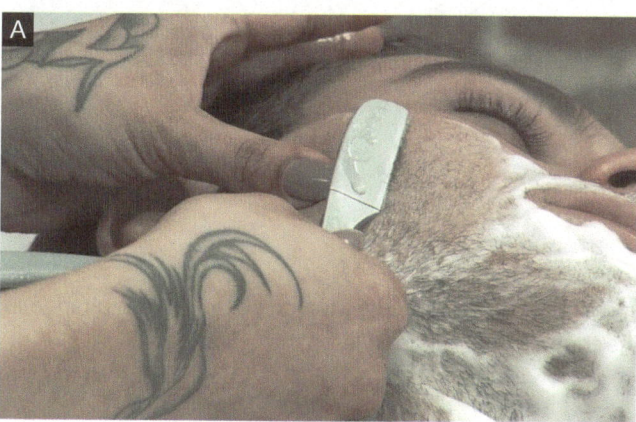
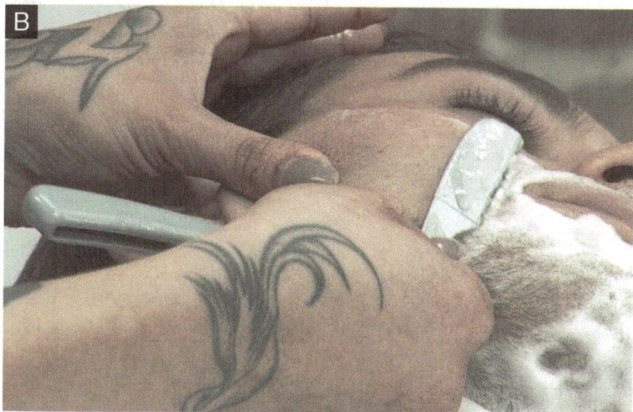

29 Stretch the skin and use a diagonal stroke from point to heel to shave the right side from the angle of the mouth to the point of the chin.

30 Wipe razor clean.

Shaving Area No. 3—Freehand stroke

31 Maintain the same body position; hold razor in freehand position.

32 To shave beneath the nostril, slightly lift the tip of the nose, taking care not to interfere with the client's breathing. Stretch the upper lip by placing the fingers of the left hand against the nose while holding the thumb below the lower corner of the lip.

PROCEDURE 5

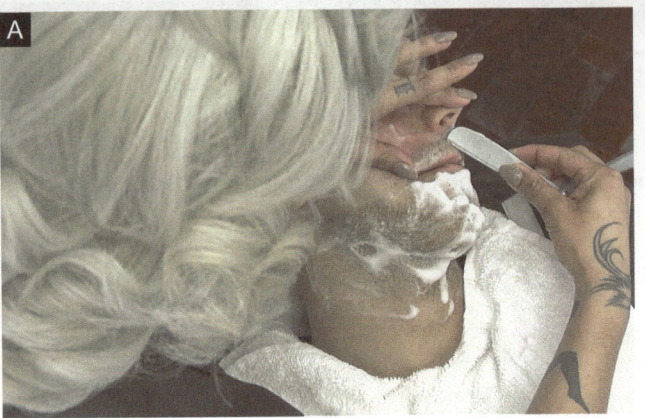
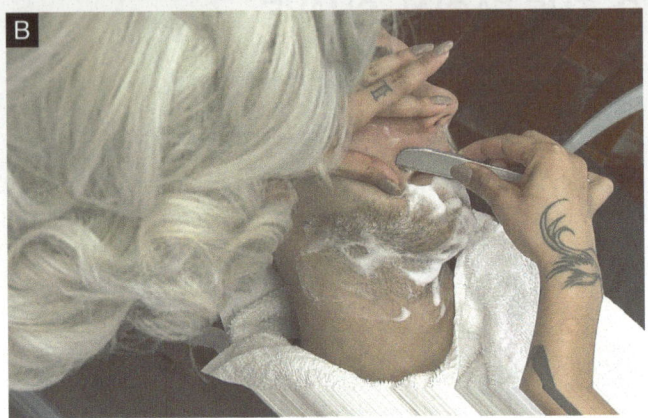

33 Shave beneath the nostrils and over the right side of the upper lip; use fingers of left hand to stretch the underlying skin. If the client wears a mustache, shave the outline with the razor at this time.

34 Wipe razor clean.

> **REMINDER**
> Shaving strokes on the upper lip are performed on a slight diagonal to follow the curves of the face; however, remember to shave *with the grain* in this area.

Shaving Area No. 4—Freehand stroke

35 Shift your body position to face the front of the right side of the client's face.

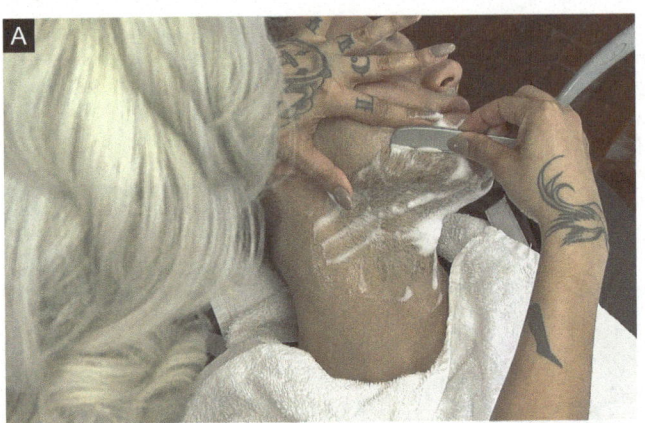
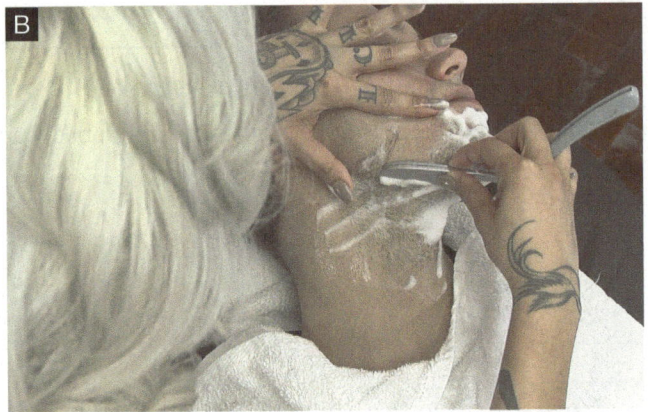

36 Starting at chin level, stretch the skin, and shave that portion of the neck below the jawbone down to the change in the grain of the beard. Be sure to hold the skin taut between the thumb and fingers of left hand.

37 Wipe razor clean.

Shaving Area No. 5—Reverse-freehand stroke

38 Move behind the chair; hold the razor for the reverse-freehand stroke.

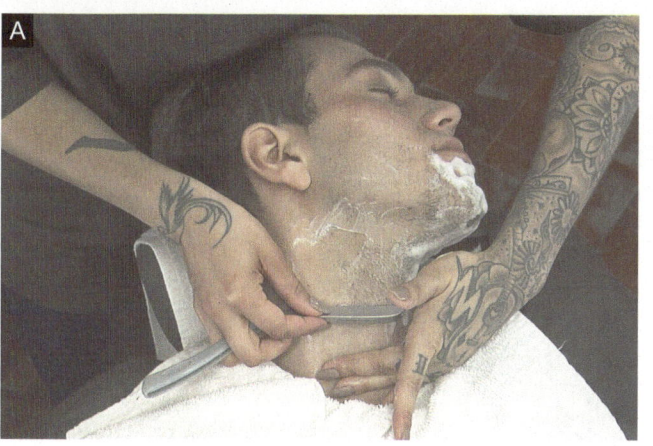
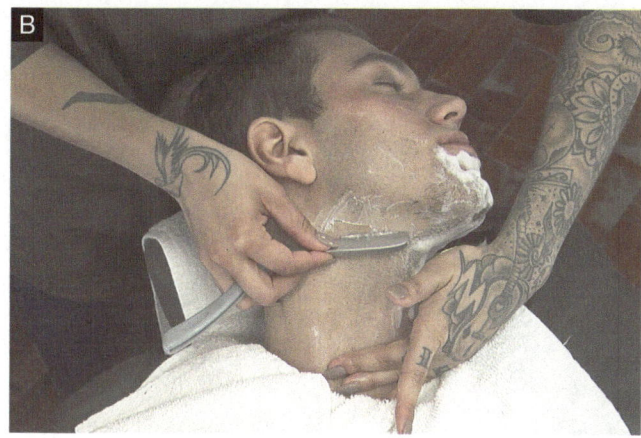

39 Stretch the skin from the bottom of Shaving Area No. 5 and shave upward with the grain. Do not expect to complete this shaving area in one stroke.

40 After completing the first stroke, reposition the razor just right of the previously shaved section until the entire area is shaved. This movement completes shaving of the right side of the face the first time over.

41 Wipe razor clean.

> **REMINDER**
> The beard should be shaved with the grain of the hair; therefore, you must determine when the reverse hand positions and strokes are the correct procedure for shaving the client's beard. For example, when the hair in Shaving Area No. 5 grows downward, the freehand stroke may be a better choice than the reverse-freehand stroke.

Shaving Area No. 6—Backhand stroke

42 Stand to the right side of the client; turn the client's face to access left upper lip. Re-lather if necessary. Hold the razor in the backhand position.

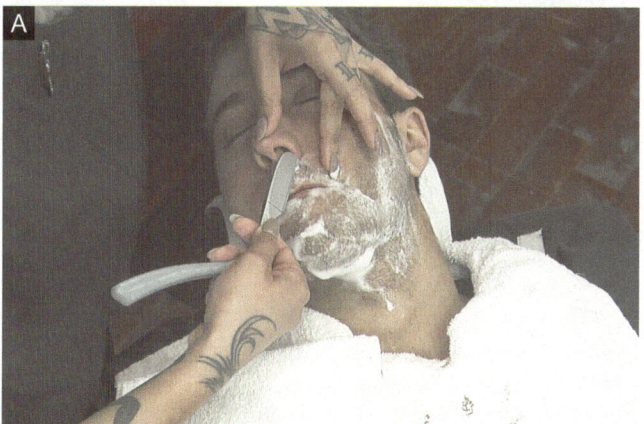
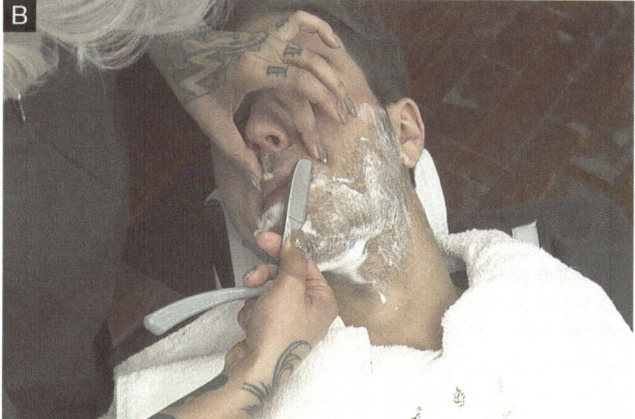

43 While gently pushing the tip of the nose to the right with the thumb and fingers of the left hand, stretch the skin and shave left side of upper lip.

44 Wipe razor clean.

PROCEDURE 5

Shaving Area No. 7—Backhand stroke

45 Move toward client's right shoulder and gently turn his face to the right. Re-lather the left side of the face.

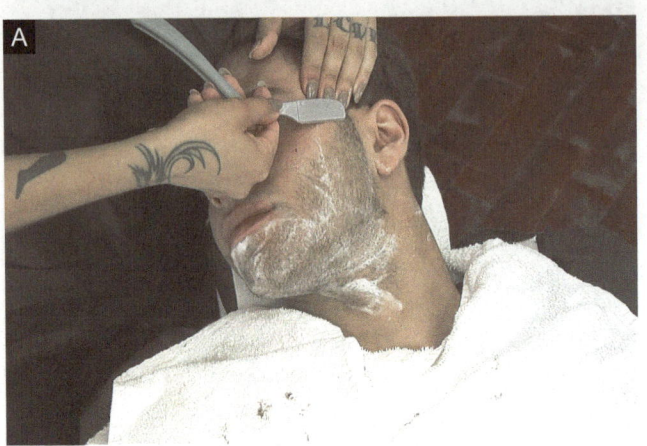
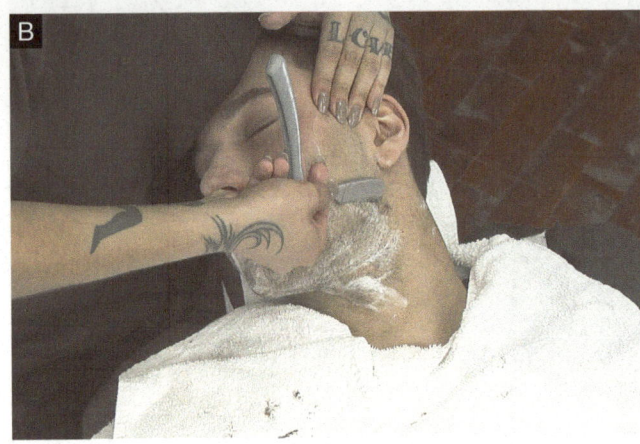

46 Using the thumb, wipe lather from the hairline. Stretch the skin taut and shave downward and slightly forward toward the corner of the mouth and jawbone.

47 Wipe razor clean.

Shaving Area No. 8—Freehand stroke

48 Stand at client's right and position his head to access this shaving area.

49 Hold razor in a freehand position.

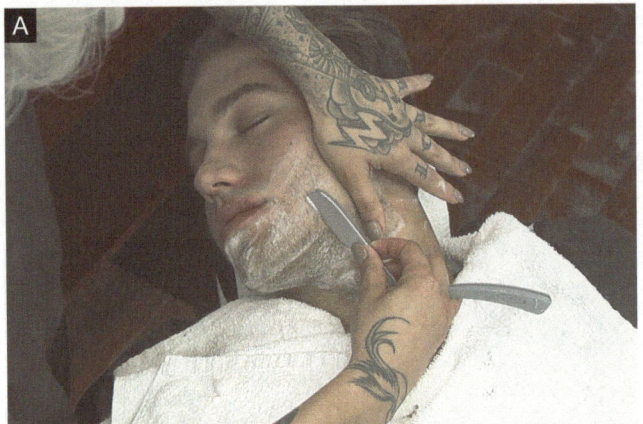
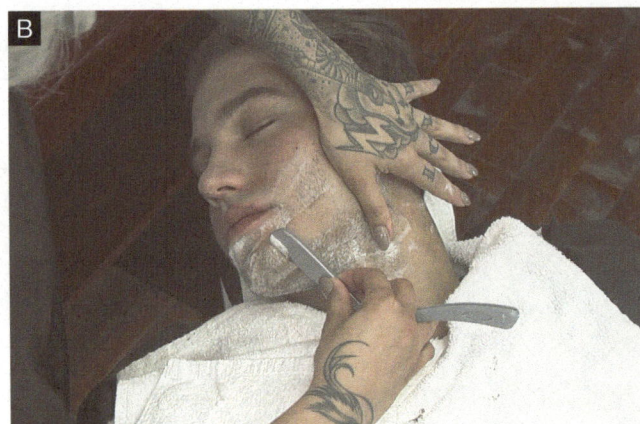

50 Stretch the skin and shave downward on the left side from the angle of the mouth to the point of the chin.

51 Wipe razor clean.

Shaving Area No. 9—Backhand stroke

52 Shift body position to access Shaving Area No. 9; hold razor for backhand stroke.

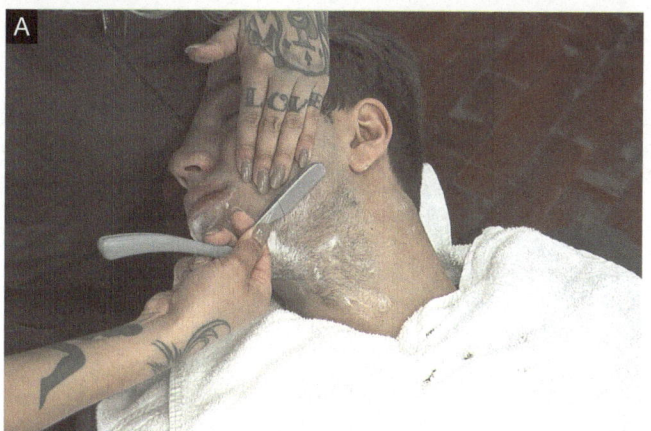 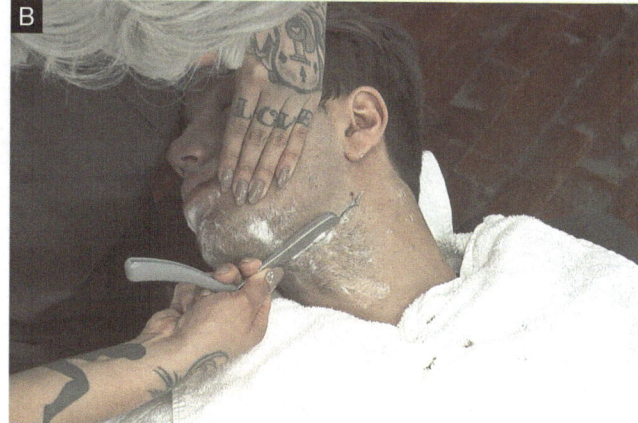

53 With the fingers of the left hand stretching the skin, shave downward from the point of the chin to where the grain of the beard changes on the neck.

54 Wipe razor clean.

Shaving Area No. 10—Reverse-freehand stroke

55 Stand behind client; hold razor in reverse-freehand position.

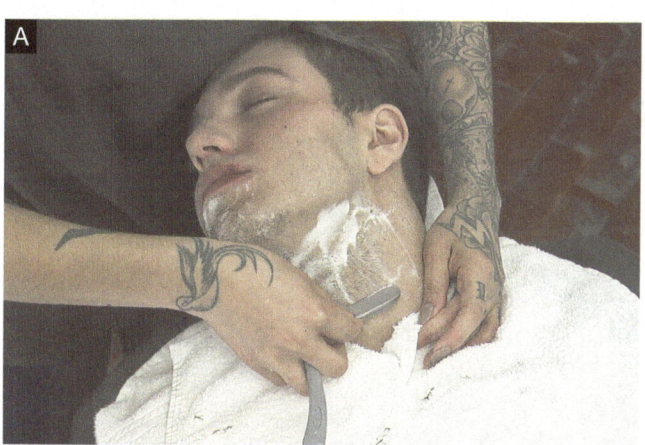 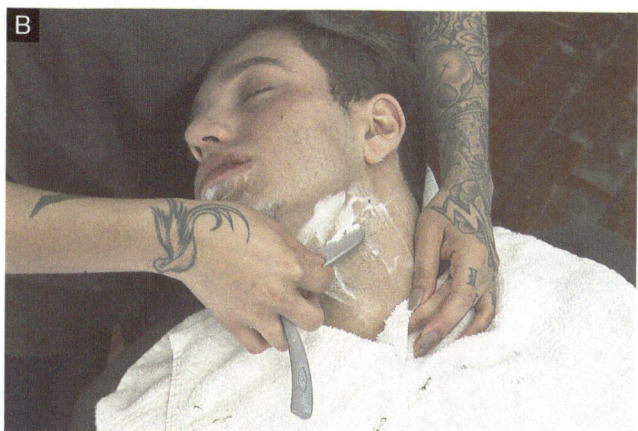

56 Stretch skin from the bottom of Shaving Area No. 10 with the left hand; shave left side of lower neck area upward to where the grain changes.

57 Similar to Shaving Area No. 5, after completing the first stroke, reposition the razor just left of the previously shaved section until the entire area is shaved. This completes the shaving of the left side of the face.

58 Wipe razor clean.

PROCEDURE 5

Shaving Area No. 11—Freehand stroke

59 Stand at the client's side; reposition his face to access Shaving Area No. 11.

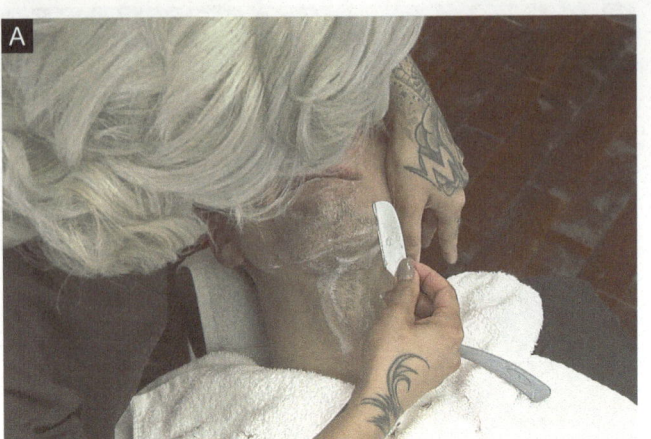
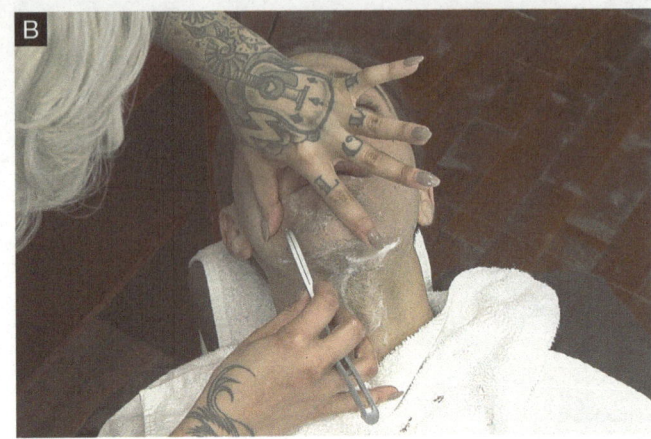

60 Hold the razor in a freehand position and stretch the skin; shave across the chin. Continue shaving until the entire chin area has been shaved to a point just below the jawbone.

61 Wipe razor clean.

> **DID YOU KNOW?**
> In Shaving Area Nos. 11 and 14, the client can help to stretch the skin if he rolls his bottom lip slightly over his bottom teeth. This is sometimes called *balling-the-chin*.

Shaving Area No. 12—Freehand or backhand stroke

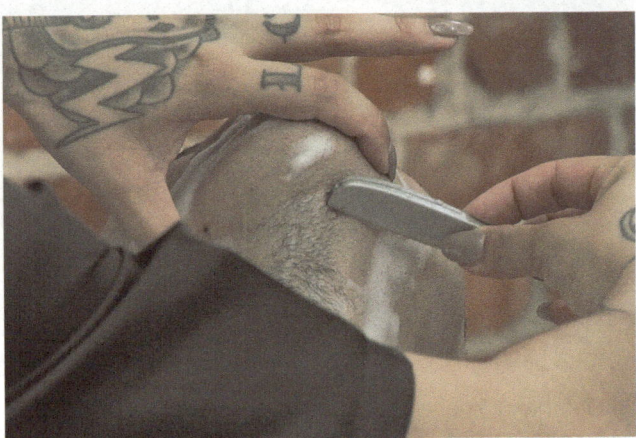
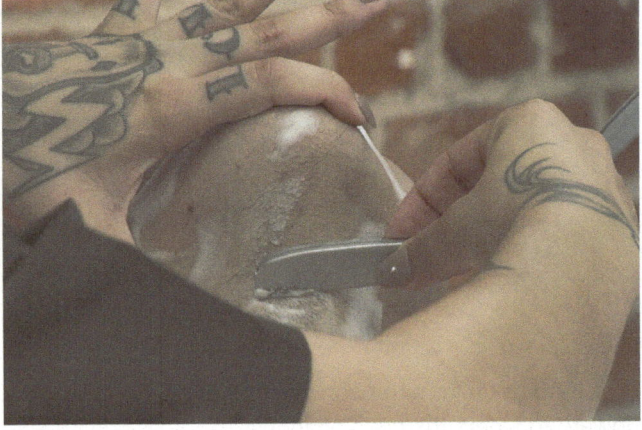

62 Using the freehand stroke, stretch the skin with the left hand and position the razor to arc downward just below the chin.

63 Continue this stroke until the grain of the beard changes.

64 Wipe razor clean.

65 Alternate method: Some professionals prefer to use the backhand stroke in Shaving Area No. 12.

PROCEDURE 5

Shaving Area No. 13—Reverse-freehand stroke

66 Stand behind the chair; hold razor for reverse-freehand stroke.

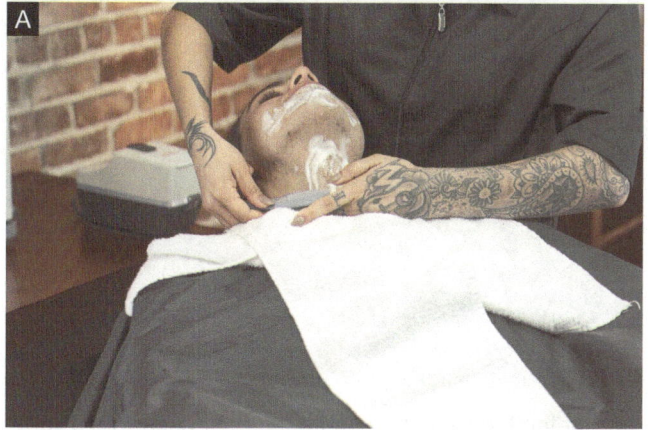
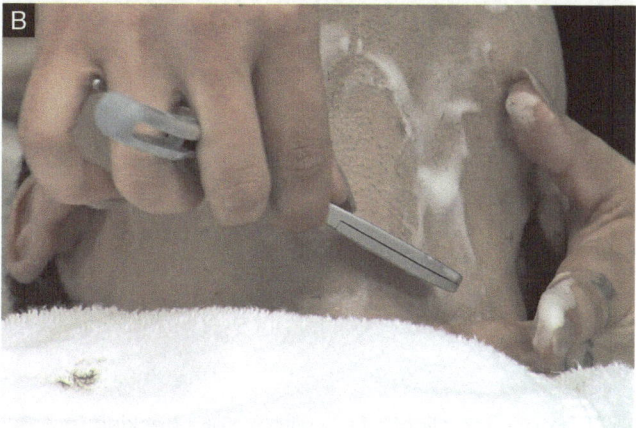

67 Stretch the skin from below Shaving Area No. 13 under the chin; shave upward on the lower part of the neck. Stretch the skin away from the Adam's apple and shave on a slight diagonal to prevent nicks.

68 Wipe razor clean.

Shaving Area No. 14—Reverse-freehand stroke

69 Remain behind the chair. Cup the client's chin and stretch the skin.

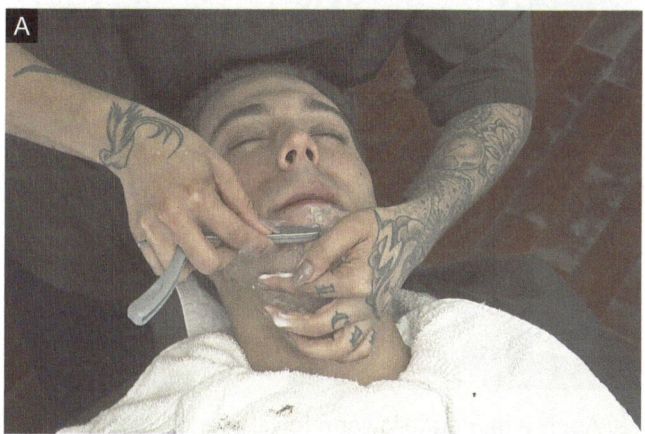
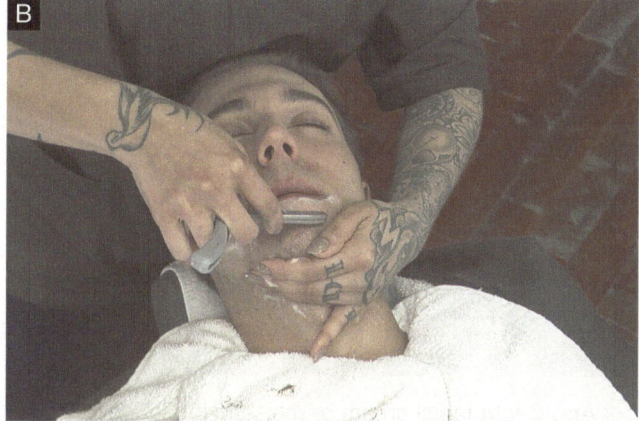

70 Using the reverse-freehand stroke, use a few short scooping strokes to shave upward from the top of the chin toward the lower lip. You may also ask the client to ball his chin for this step.

71 Wipe the razor clean and discard the towel or paper strip. This completes the first-time-over shave procedure.

MILADY STANDARD SHAVING

PROCEDURE 5

Second-Time-Over Shave

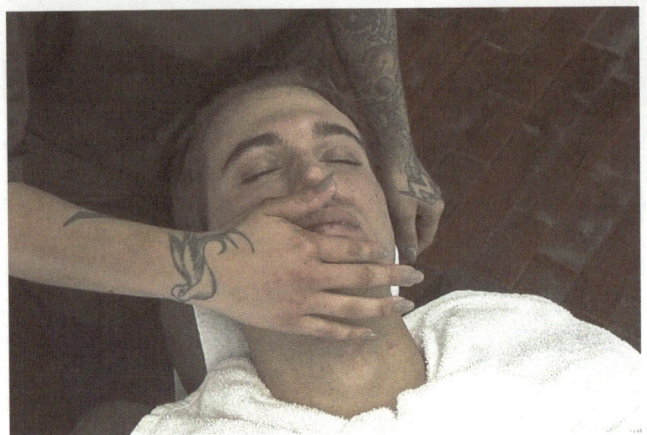

72 Dampen the client's face with water, checking for rough or uneven spots as you moisten the skin.

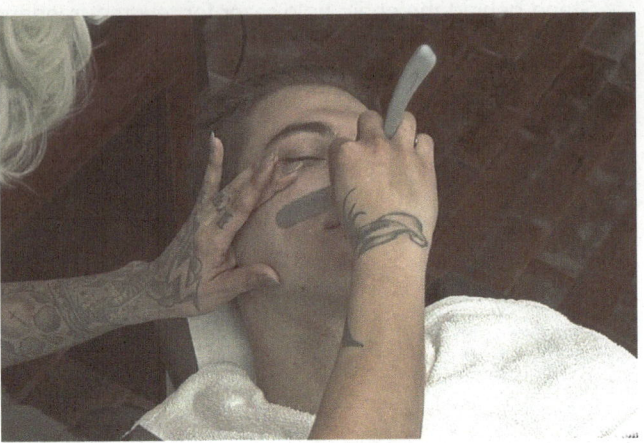

73 Stretch the skin and use freehand strokes with a light touch to shave with or across the grain to remove any residual facial hair.

74 Remove and dispose of wiping towel or paper. Lay a clean towel across client's chest.

D. FINISHING STEPS OF THE SHAVE

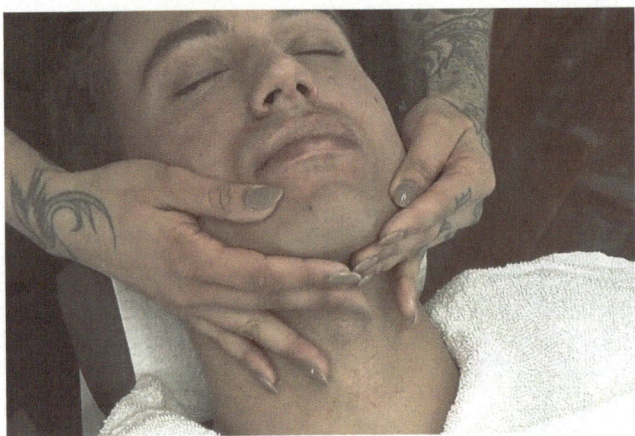

75 Apply light facial cream or moisturizing lotion with an effleurage massage movement. Massage the cream into the skin using pétrissage massage movements.

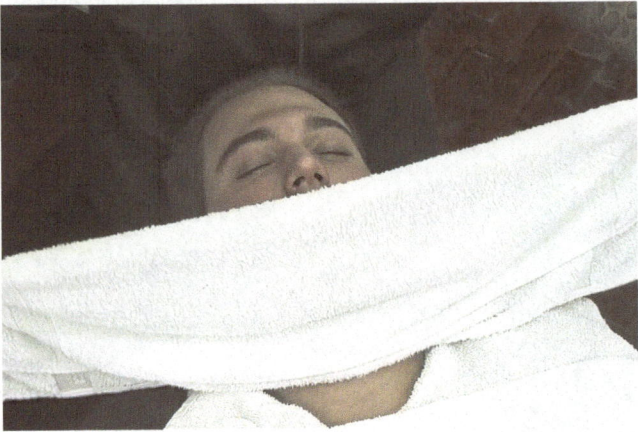

76 Apply a moderately warm towel over client's face.

77 Remove the towel and wipe off excess product in one operation.

> ⚠ **CAUTION**
> Avoid hot towels as the skin may be sensitive after the shave service.

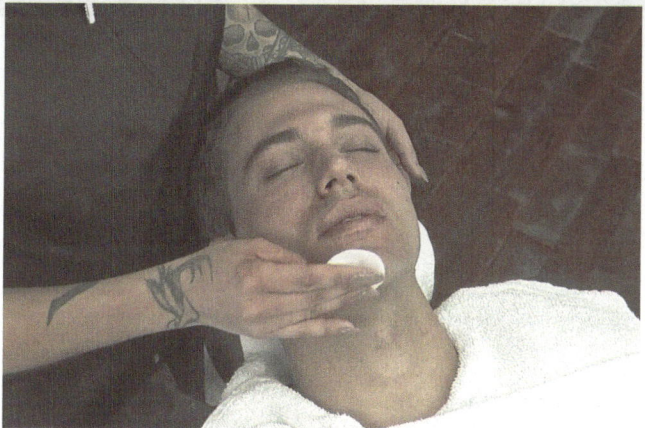

78 Apply a skin toner or other mild astringent using cotton pledgets or a soft tissue to remove residual cream product. Pat gently; do not wipe or scrape against the skin.

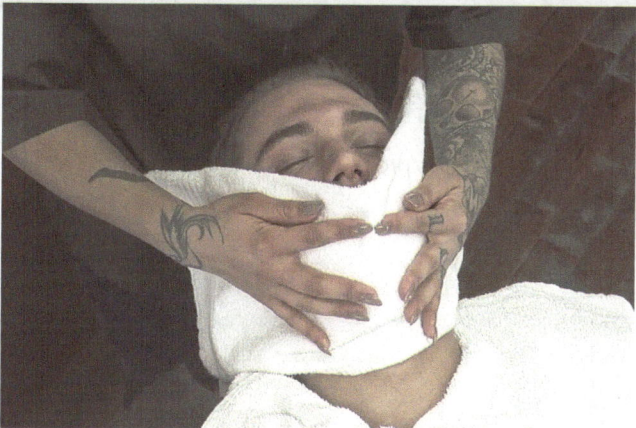

79 Remove the towel from the client's chest and position yourself behind the chair. Spread the towel over the client's face. Pat dry the lower part of the face; then the upper part. Remove the towel and fan the face dry.

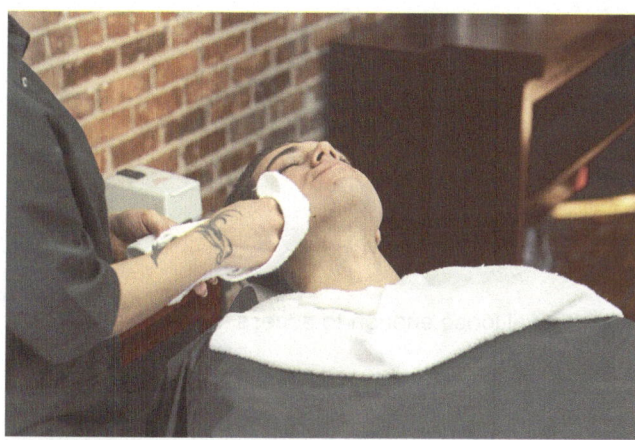

80 Move to the side of the chair and wrap a clean dry towel around your hand. Sprinkle a small amount of talcum powder on the towel and apply evenly to the face, if desired by client.

81 Slowly return the client to a sitting position.

82 Offer to perform a neck shave.

83 Comb the hair neatly as desired.

84 Wipe off loose hair, lather, or powder from the client's face, neck, and clothing. Proceed with mustache trim, if not performed before shave service, or neck shave, as desired. Remove draping.

CLEAN-UP AND DISINFECTION

- ☐ Clean and disinfect the tools and implements.
- ☐ Clean and then disinfect the work area.
- ☐ Sweep up hair and deposit in a closed receptacle.
- ☐ Deposit used blades in a sharps container.
- ☐ Dispose of single-use items. Place all used linens, towels, and capes in the laundry.
- ☐ Wash your hands.

P-6

THE NECK SHAVE

After practicing this procedure, you should be able to:

LO 15 Demonstrate a neck shave.

MATERIALS, IMPLEMENTS, AND EQUIPMENT

- ☐ Barber chair
- ☐ Comb and brush
- ☐ Covered container for soiled towels
- ☐ Covered trash can
- ☐ Electric latherizer
- ☐ Haircutting cape
- ☐ Paper towels
- ☐ Sharps container
- ☐ Shaving cream or gel
- ☐ Sink
- ☐ Straight razor and blades
- ☐ Terry cloth towels
- ☐ Witch hazel or antiseptic

PREPARATION

1. Assemble supplies.
2. Following the facial shave, raise the chair slowly to an upright position.
3. Wash your hands.
4. Tuck a towel around the back of the neck, leaving the cape and towel loose enough to access the sides and bottom of the neckline.

PROCEDURE

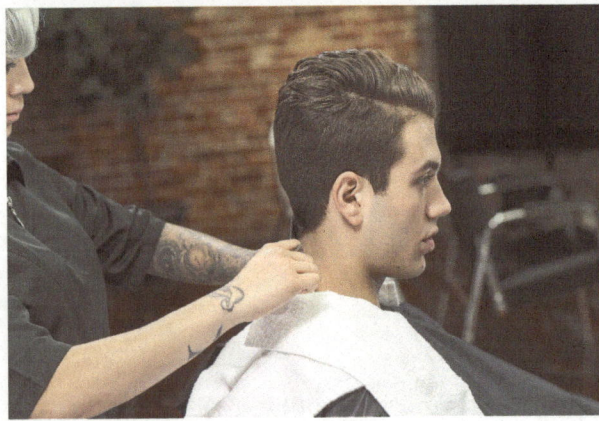

1. Tuck neck strip or paper towel into the neckline of drape for wiping the razor. Check the neckline and behind-the-ear areas for moles, blemishes, or other conditions.

PROCEDURE 6

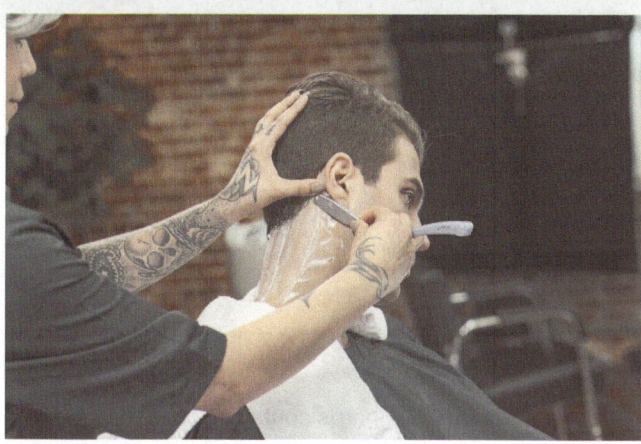

② Apply lather. Stretch the skin behind the right ear with the thumb and shave along the natural hairline down the side of the neck using a freehand stroke.

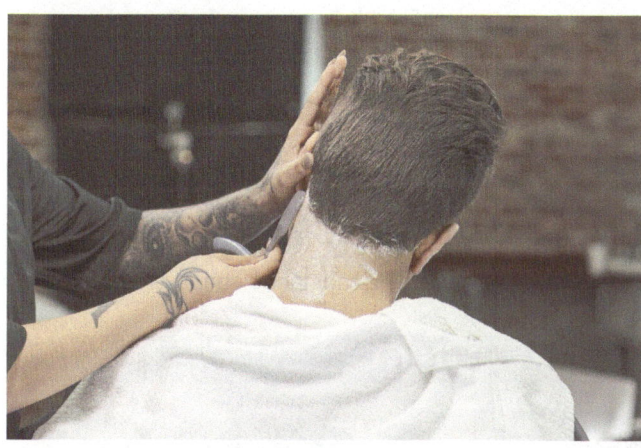

③ Repeat on left side using a reverse-backhand stroke.

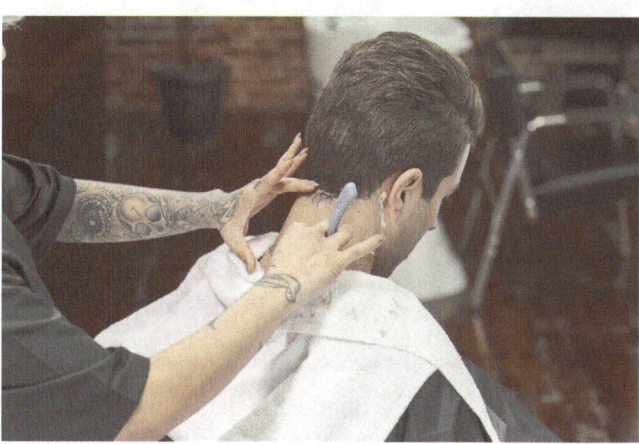

④ Use a freehand stroke to shave the nape area. Clean the shaven part of the neckline with a towel or neck strip moistened with witch hazel, antiseptic, or warm water. Remove the towel from around the neck and dry thoroughly.

⑤ Stand behind the chair, place a clean dry towel around the client's neck, and comb or style the hair as desired by the client.

⑥ Take the towel from the back of the neck and fold it around the right hand. Remove all traces of powder and any loose hair.

⑦ Discard the towel and remove the chair cloth from the client.

CLEAN-UP AND DISINFECTION

☐ Clean and disinfect the tools and implements.
☐ Clean and then disinfect the work area.
☐ Sweep up hair and deposit in a closed receptacle.
☐ Deposit used blades in a sharps container.
☐ Dispose of single-use items. Place all used linens, towels, and capes in the laundry.
☐ Wash your hands.

MILADY STANDARD SHAVING

MUSTACHE TRIM

After practicing this procedure, you should be able to:

LO 16 Demonstrate a mustache trim.

MATERIALS, IMPLEMENTS, AND EQUIPMENT

- ☐ Barber chair with headrest
- ☐ Comb and brush
- ☐ Covered container for soiled towels
- ☐ Covered trash can
- ☐ Electric latherizer
- ☐ Haircutting cape
- ☐ Haircutting shears
- ☐ Headrest cover
- ☐ Outliner or trimmer
- ☐ Paper towels
- ☐ Sharps container
- ☐ Shaving cream or gel
- ☐ Sink
- ☐ Straight razor and blades
- ☐ Terry cloth towels

PREPARATION

1. Assemble supplies.
2. Wash your hands.
3. Drape the client as for a haircut service.
4. Consult with the client regarding mustache shape preferences.

PROCEDURE

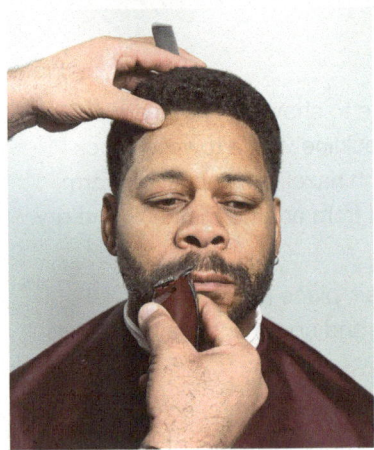

1. Trim the mustache to desired length with an outliner. Check for evenness of length at the corners of the mouth.

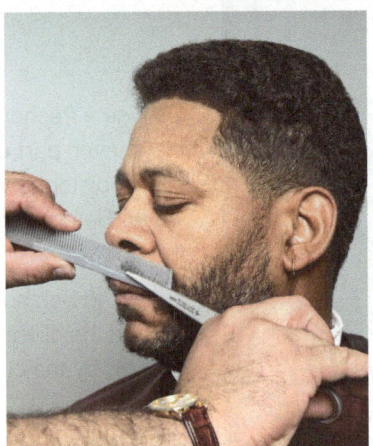

2. For safety, remove bulk from the mustache using the shear-over-comb or outliner-over-comb technique.

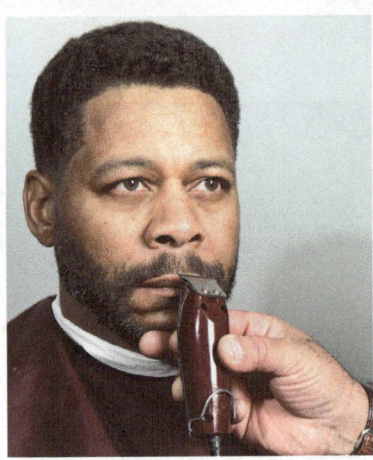

3. Shape and detail mustache with an outliner or razor. If using a razor, apply shaving cream or gel, wipe off excess product with thumb or finger, and proceed with razor outlining.

CLEAN-UP AND DISINFECTION

- ☐ Clean and disinfect the tools and implements.
- ☐ Clean and then disinfect the work area.
- ☐ Sweep up hair and deposit in a closed receptacle.
- ☐ Deposit used blades in a sharps container.
- ☐ Dispose of single-use items. Place all used linens, towels, and capes in the laundry.
- ☐ Wash your hands.

P-8

BEARD DESIGNS

After practicing this procedure, you should be able to:

LO17 Demonstrate cutting in beard designs.

MATERIALS, IMPLEMENTS, AND EQUIPMENT

- ☐ Barber chair with headrest
- ☐ Clippers
- ☐ Comb and brush
- ☐ Covered container for soiled towels
- ☐ Covered trash can
- ☐ Electric latherizer
- ☐ Haircutting cape
- ☐ Haircutting shears
- ☐ Headrest cover
- ☐ Outliner or trimmer
- ☐ Paper towels
- ☐ Sharps container
- ☐ Shaving cream or gel
- ☐ Sink
- ☐ Straight razor and blades
- ☐ Terry cloth towels

PREPARATION

1. Assemble supplies.
2. Wash your hands.
3. Drape the client as for a haircut service.
4. Consult with the client as to his desired design of the beard. Determine any preferences regarding length, density (thickness), and shape.

> **HERE'S A TIP**
> A cloth towel is a good alternative to a neck strip, especially if the client has a lot of hair growth on his neck.

PROCEDURE

A. BEARD TRIM ON MEDIUM-TEXTURED FACIAL HAIR

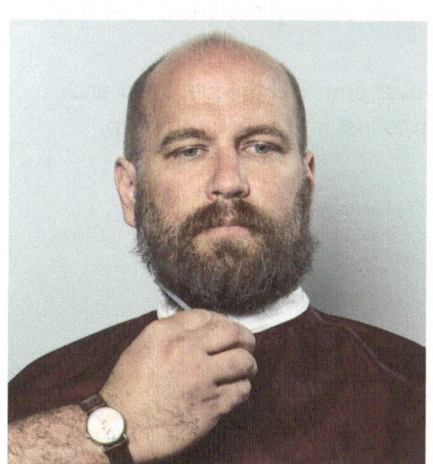

1. Gently comb through the beard and check for hidden moles or growths.

2. Apply a fresh headrest cover. Adjust the headrest so the client's neck is supported while leaning his head back. The chair back may also be reclined at a slight angle, depending on your preference for reaching areas under the chin. Place a towel underneath the chin to protect the client's neck from stray hairs (optional).

PROCEDURE 8

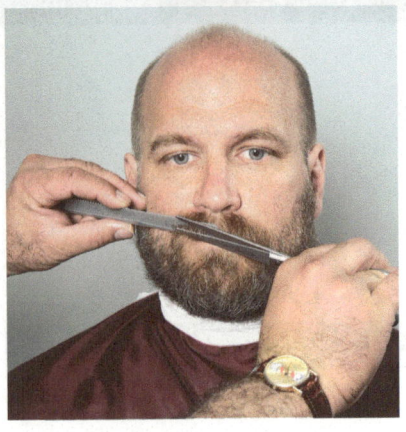

③ Trim excess mustache hair using the shear-over-comb or clipper-over-comb technique.

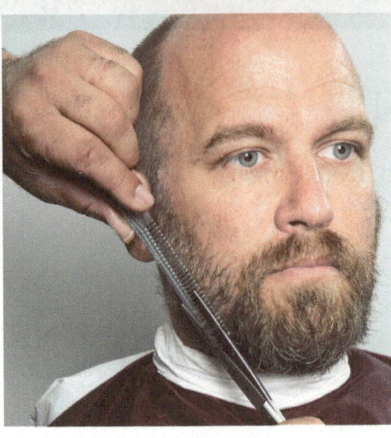

④ Trim excess hair in cheek areas.

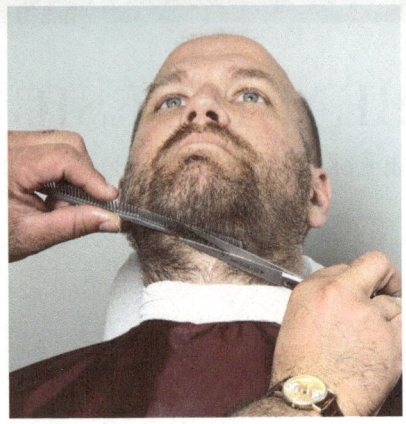

⑤ Trim excess hair under chin.

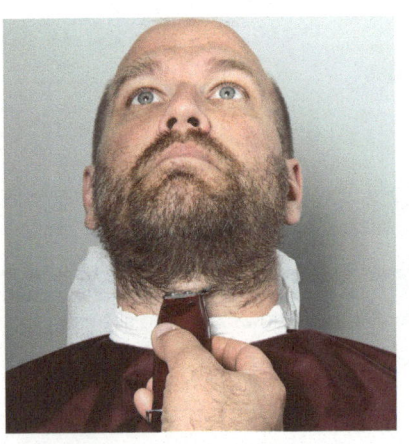

⑥ Start in the center directly under the chin and establish a guide with the outliner.

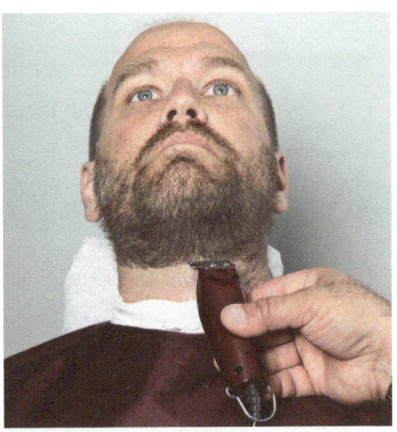

⑦ Work left and right of center to establish design line to back of the jaws.

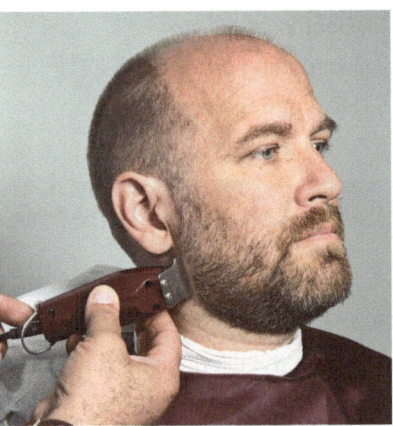

⑧ Move to the client's right side and cut in the design from the sideburn down to the guide at the back of the jaw. Repeat on the left side.

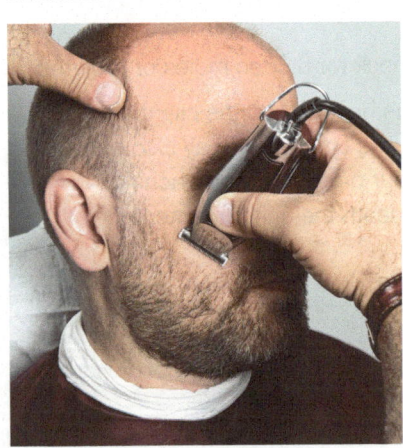

⑨ Use trimmer to outline the cheek and upper areas of the beard, blending with the sideburn area.

⑩ Using the shear-over-comb or clipper-over-comb technique, taper and blend the beard from the outlined areas up to just under the bottom lip, mustache, and cheek areas.

PROCEDURE 8

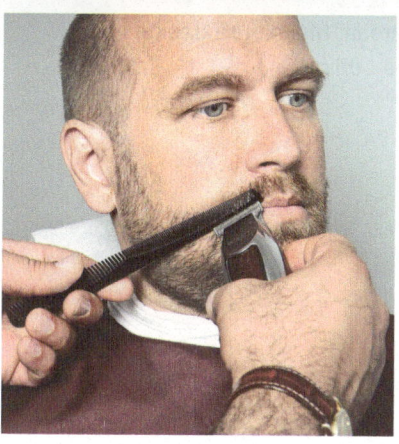

11 Trim and blend the mustache into the beard using the shear-, clipper-, or outliner-over-comb technique.

12 Recline client, apply steam towel, lather areas to be shaved, shave carefully at the outline, and wipe clean. Apply aftershave or tonic lotion.

13 Return client to sitting position.

14 Remember to check the proportion and shape of the beard in the mirror when the client is returned to a sitting position. Retouch the beard design with shears or outliner wherever necessary.

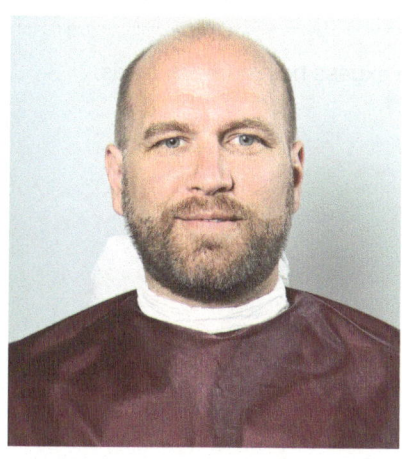

15 Style or cut the hair as needed for a finished look.

B. BEARD REDESIGN ON MEDIUM-TEXTURED FACIAL HAIR

The following steps show the procedure for creating a new mustache and beard design starting from the trim just performed.

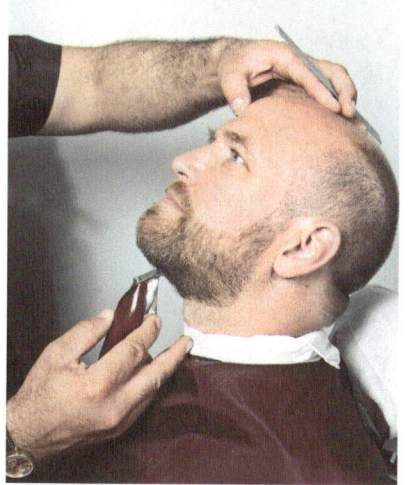

16 Use outliner to create a new guide starting in the center under the chin.

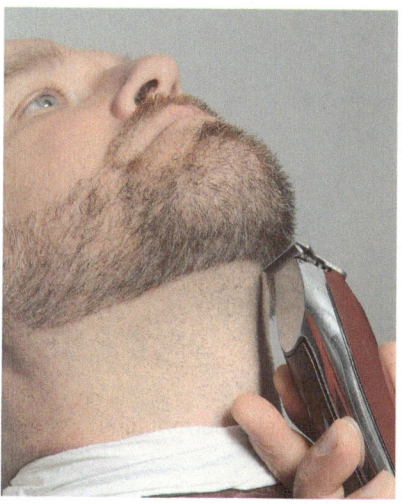

17 Cut right and left of center to establish new design line.

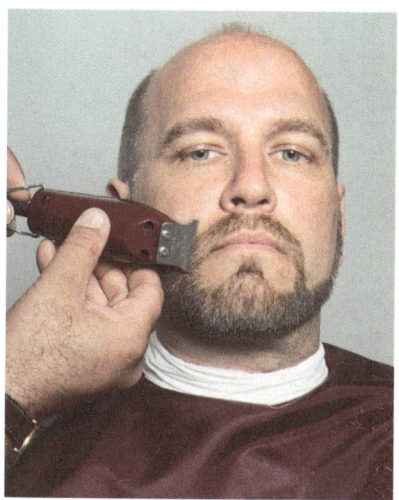

18 Reshape mustache and chin areas.

MILADY STANDARD SHAVING 53

PROCEDURE 8

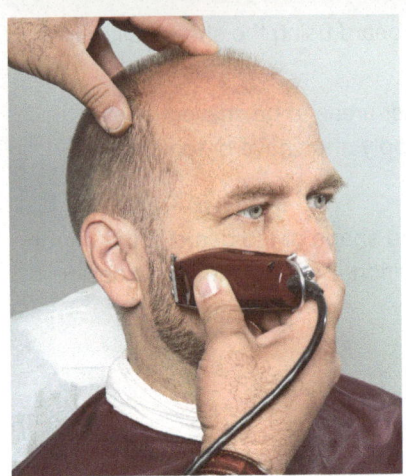

19 Cut in a new design line in the cheek areas. Make sure design line connects with the corners of the mustache outline.

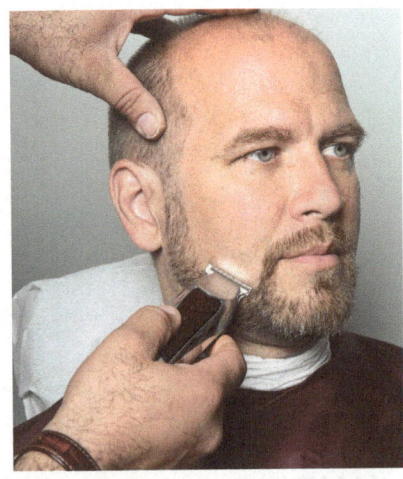

20 With outliner blades facing up, remove excess hair in cheek areas.

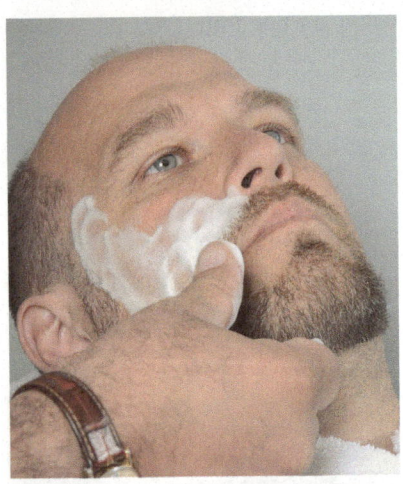

21 Recline client and apply shaving cream along new outlines.

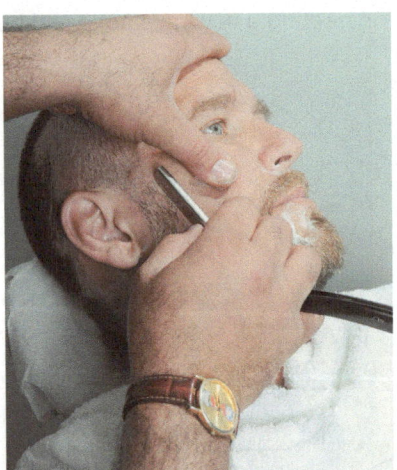

22 Shave sideburn outline.

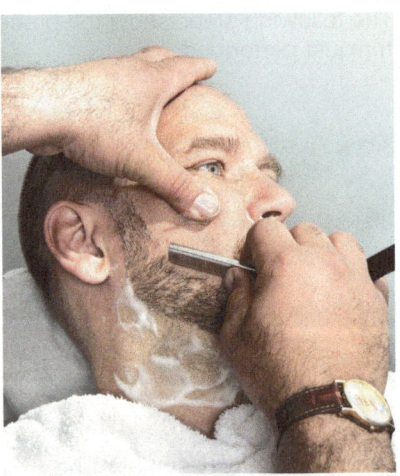

23 Shave cheek outline.

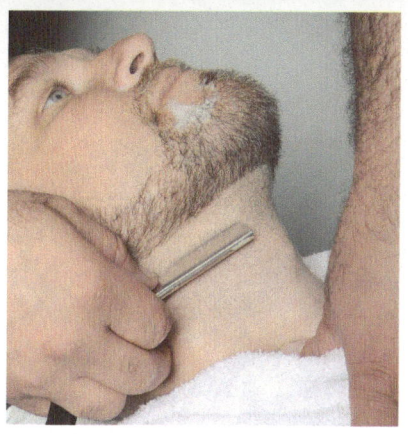
24 Shave neck areas 5 and 10.

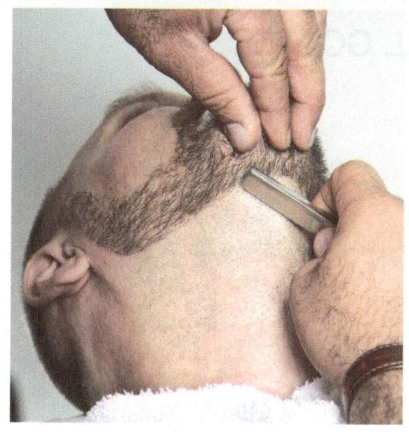
25 Shave neck areas 12 and 13.

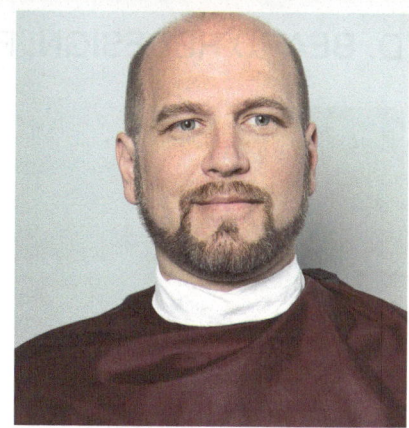
26 Finish design.

C. BEARD TRIM ON CURLY-TEXTURED FACIAL HAIR

Note: This procedure shows the progression of three designs from a full beard to a patch and goatee.

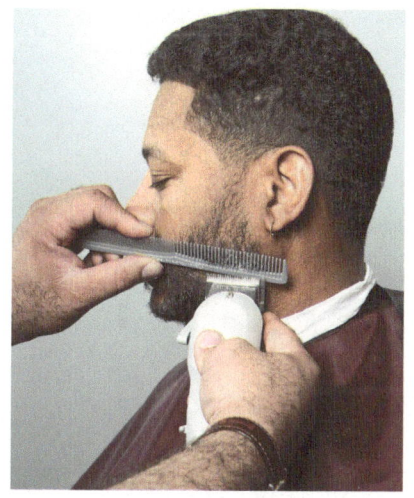
27 Trim excess hair using the clipper-over-comb technique.

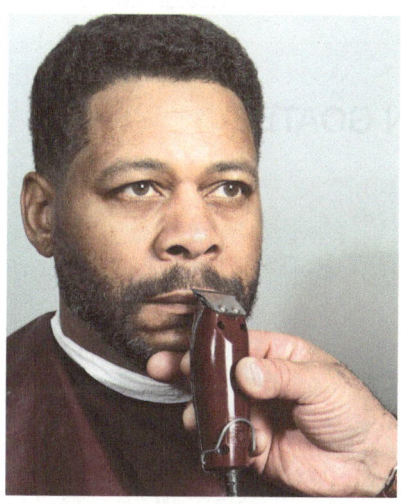
28 Trim and shape mustache.

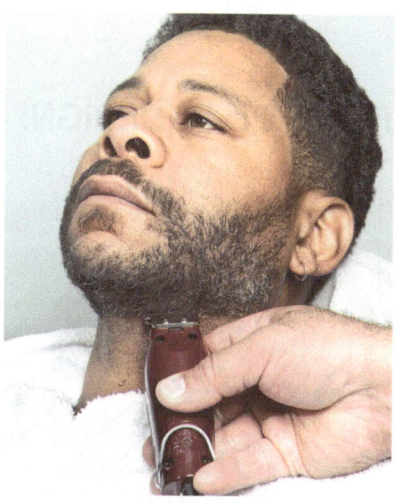
29 Establish design line under chin.

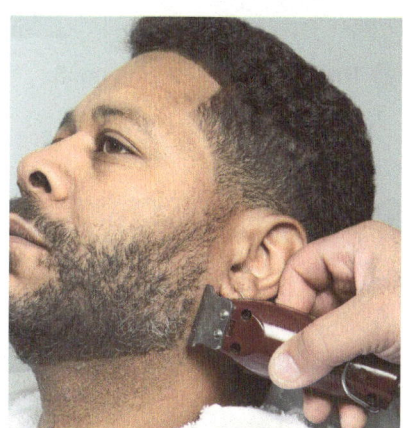
30 Establish design line at jaw and sideburn areas.

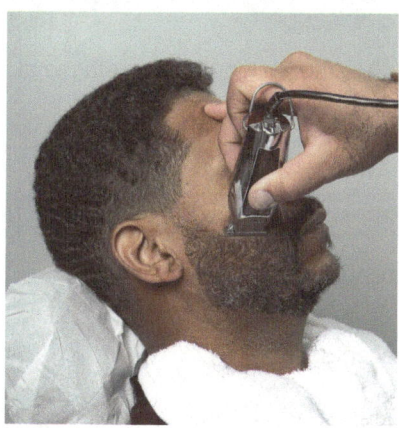
31 Establish design line in cheek areas.

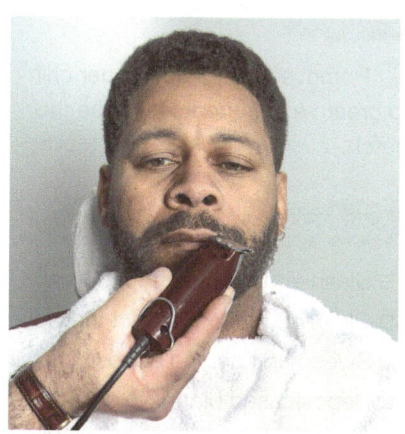
32 Contour under mustache above top lip. This completes design no. 1.

D. BEARD REDESIGN: FULL GOATEE

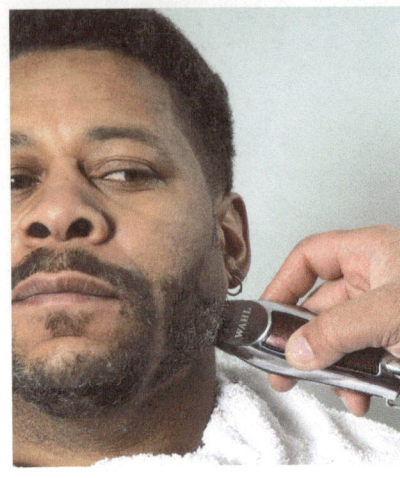

33 Remove cheek and side hair to create a full goatee.

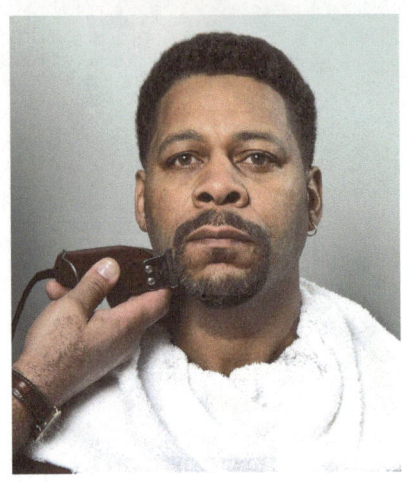

34 Contour full goatee design line. This completes design no. 2.

E. BEARD REDESIGN: CHIN GOATEE

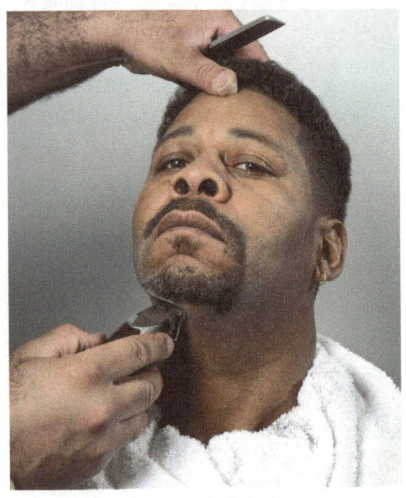

35 Remove excess hair under chin to create a chin goatee; shape the patch.

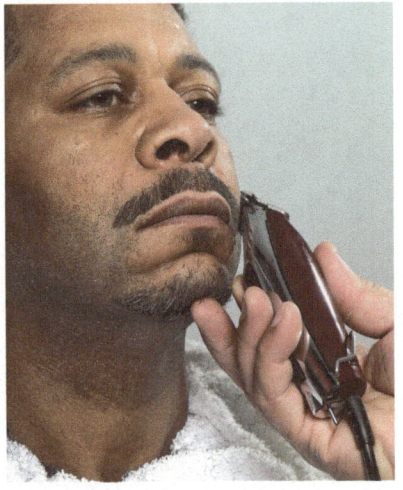

36 Establish length of mustache at corners.

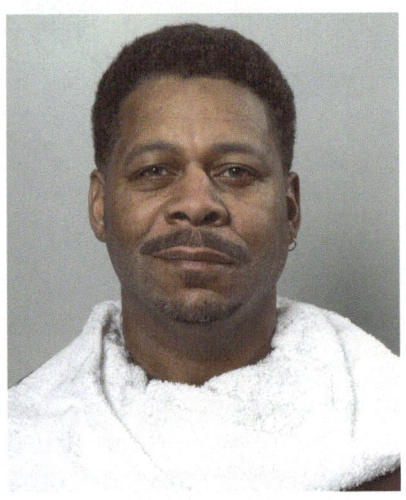

37 This completes design no. 3.

CLEAN-UP AND DISINFECTION

☐ Clean and disinfect the tools and implements.
☐ Clean and then disinfect the work area.
☐ Sweep up hair and deposit in a closed receptacle.
☐ Deposit used blades in a sharps container.
☐ Dispose of single-use items. Place all used linens, towels, and capes in the laundry.
☐ Wash your hands.

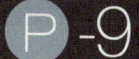

ARCHING TECHNIQUE WITH RAZOR

> **HERE'S A TIP**
> Before beginning **arching** (ARE-ching), check to determine if one sideburn is longer than the other. Start on the side with the shorter sideburn to avoid unnecessary repetition of the procedure.

MATERIALS, IMPLEMENTS, AND EQUIPMENT

- ☐ All-purpose comb
- ☐ Haircutting cape
- ☐ Neck strips
- ☐ Razor and blade

PREPARATION

1. Wash your hands.
2. Conduct a client consultation.
3. Drape the client for the haircut service.
4. Face the client toward the mirror and lock the chair.

PROCEDURE

ARCHING TECHNIQUE WITH RAZOR

1. Apply shaving cream to the bottom of the sideburn and around the ear.

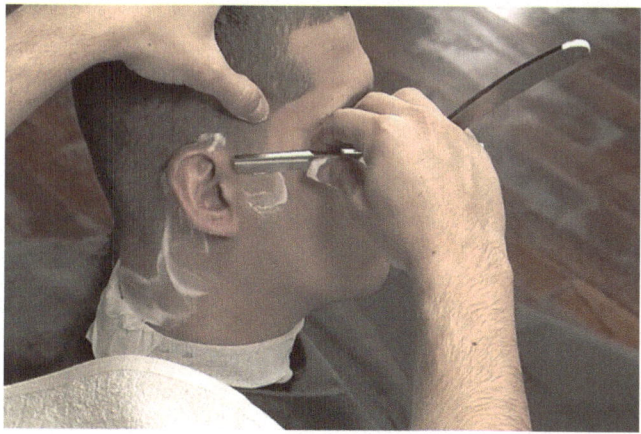

2. Shave the bottom of the sideburn using the freehand stroke.

MILADY STANDARD SHAVING 57

PROCEDURE 9

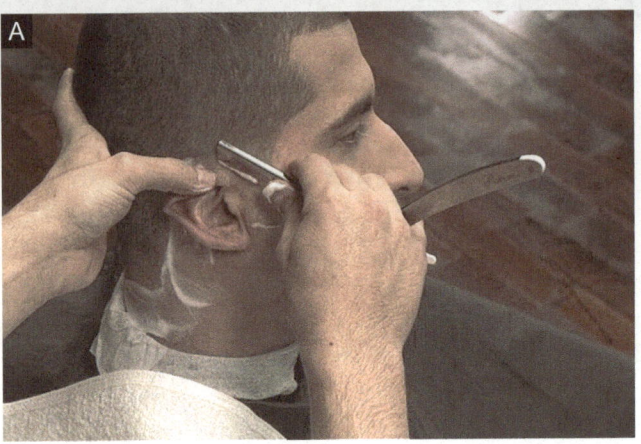 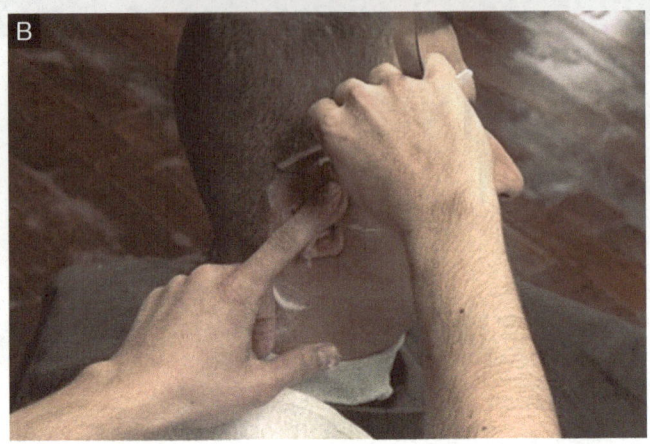

③ Gently bend or fold the ear out of the way to shave at the hairline in front of and over the ear.

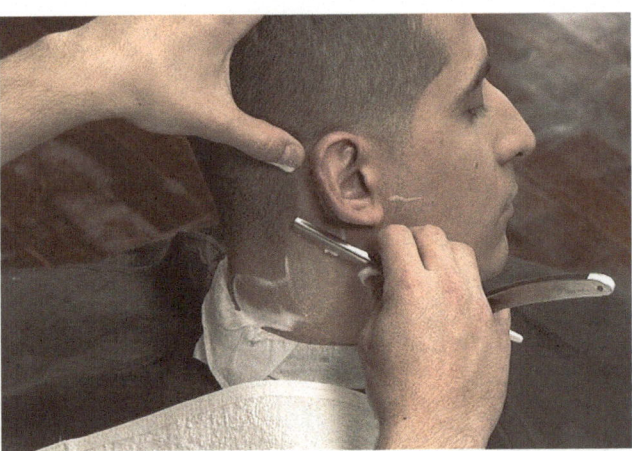

④ Shave in back of the ear to the corner of the nape.

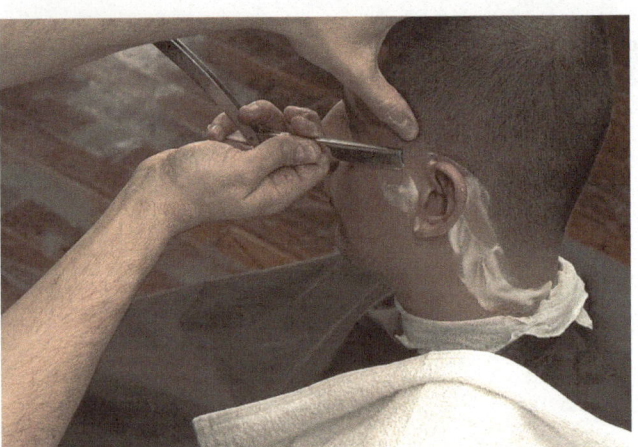

⑤ Repeat the procedure on the left side, using the backhand and reverse backhand strokes.

58   MILADY STANDARD SHAVING

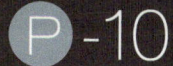

OUTLINE SHAVE

Note: An outline shave involves shaving the bottom of the sideburns, around and behind the ears, the nape area, and, when appropriate for the hairstyle, the front hairline. This procedure provides the steps for a complete outline shave.

MATERIALS, IMPLEMENTS, AND EQUIPMENT

- ☐ Disposable towels
- ☐ Haircutting cape
- ☐ Neck strips
- ☐ Shaving cream or gel
- ☐ Straight razor and blades
- ☐ Terry cloth towels

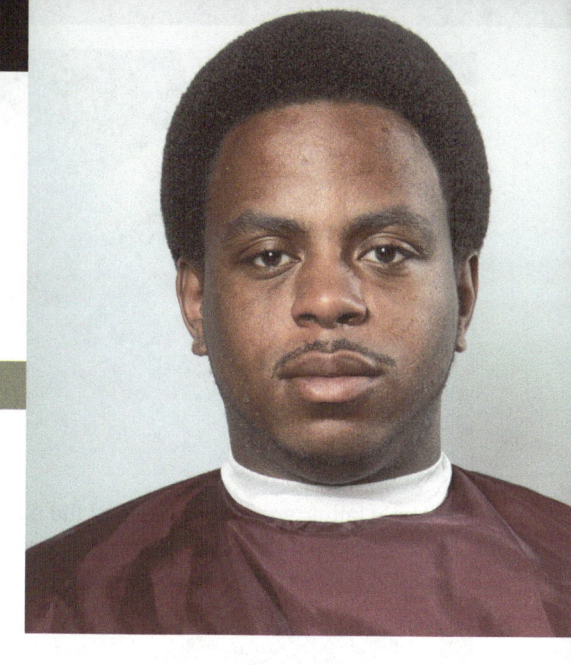

PREPARATION

1. Client should still be draped from the haircut service.
2. Disinfect razor and blades.
3. Wash your hands.
4. Loosen the cape and apply towel to neckline, leaving it loose enough for access to the nape when securing the drape.

PROCEDURE

1. Apply a light coating of lather at the front hairline.

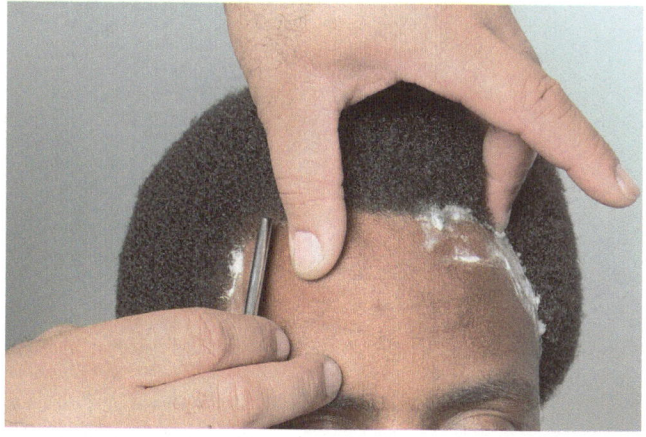

2. Stand at a slight diagonal to the client. Stretch the skin at the forehead and shave from the center along the front hairline to the temple area using the freehand stroke.

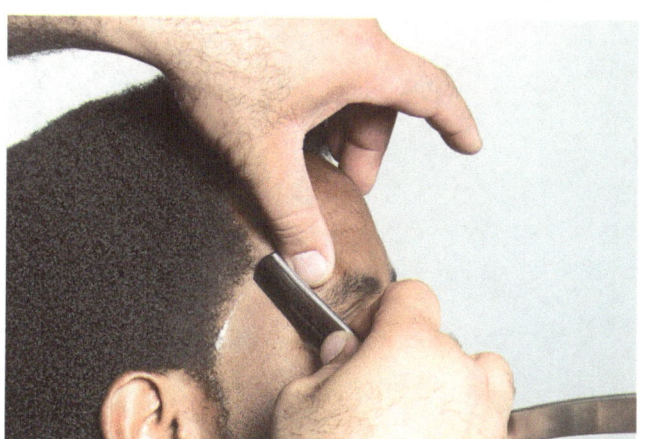

3. Shave from the temple along the hairline to the front of the sideburn.

MILADY STANDARD SHAVING

PROCEDURE 10

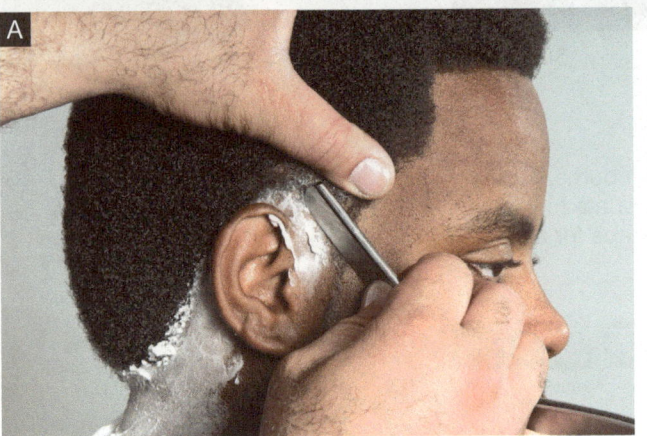
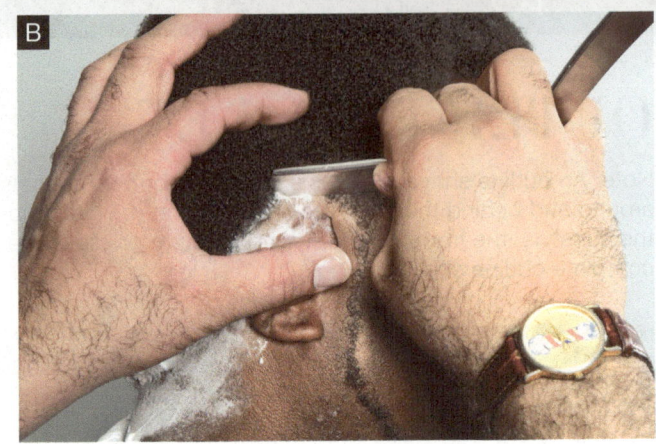

4 Apply lather around and behind the ear. Using the freehand stroke, begin shaving in front of the ear; then hold the ear away and shave around the ear.

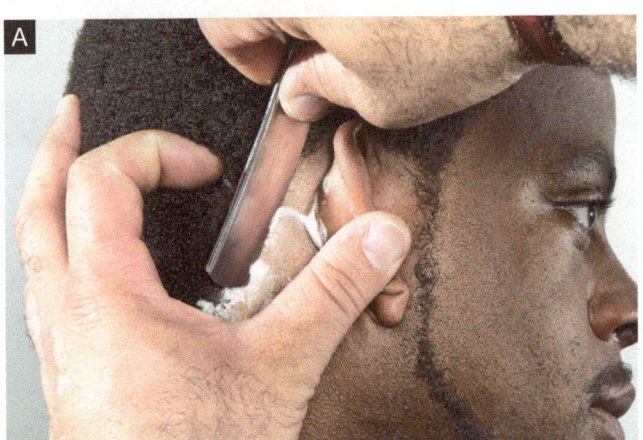
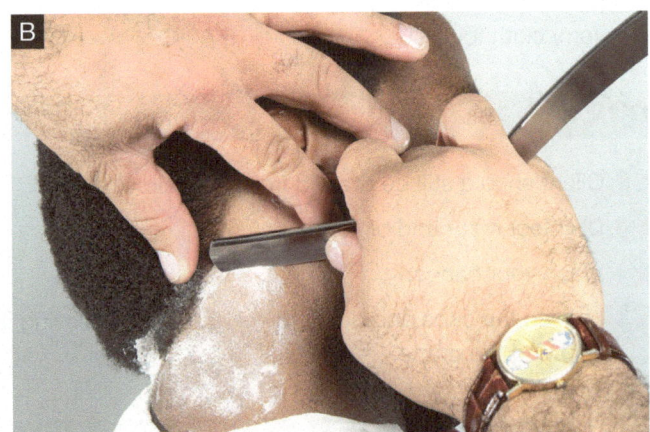

5 Shave behind the ear and down the side of the neck using the freehand stroke.

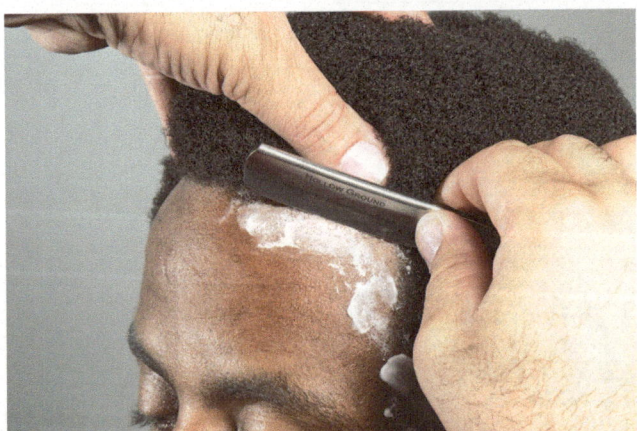
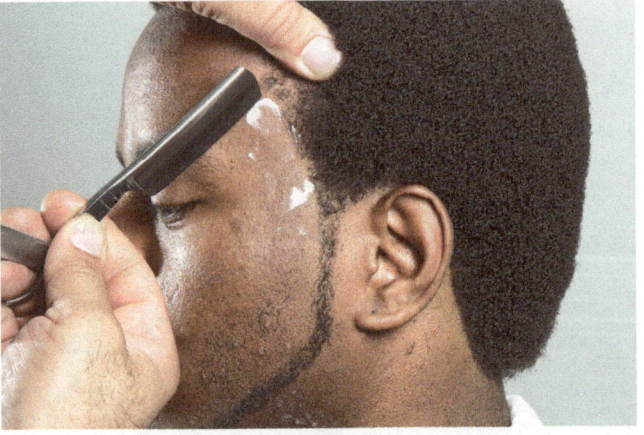

6 Move to the client's left side and reapply lather at forehead. Stretch the skin at the forehead area and repeat freehand strokes to the temple.

7 Use the backhand stroke to shave from the temple to the front sideburn area.

PROCEDURE 10

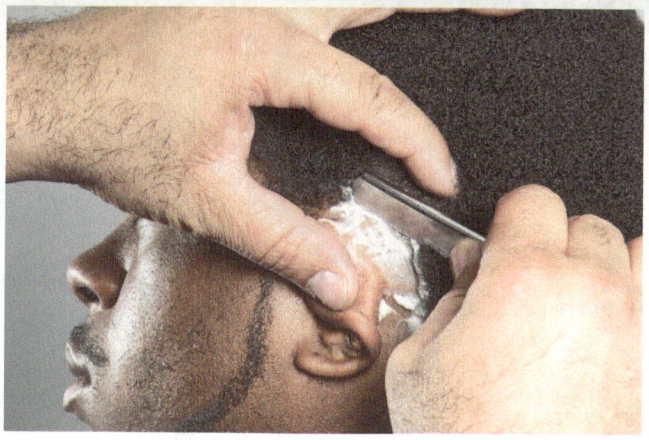 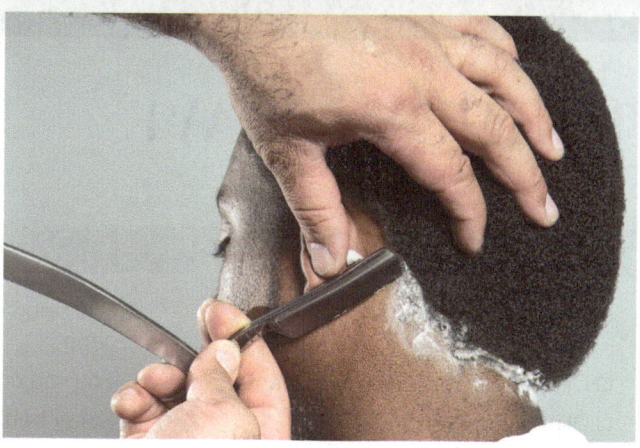

8 Apply lather around and behind the ear. Use the freehand stroke to shave in front of and around the ear at the hairline, holding the ear away with the fingers.

9 Use the reverse backhand stroke to shave behind the ear and down the side of the neck.

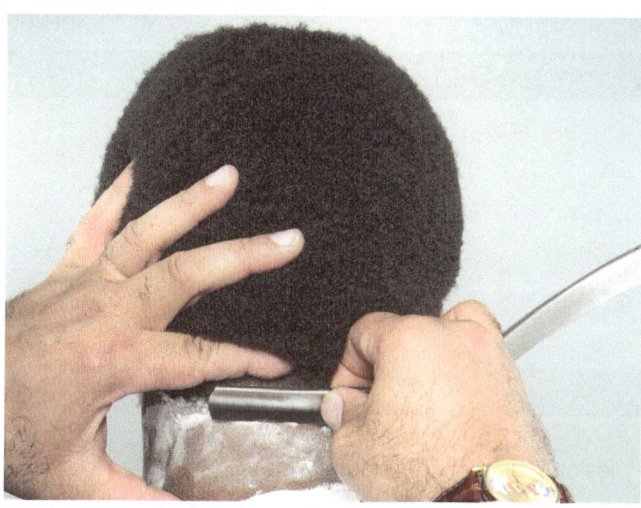

10 Shave the nape area with a freehand stroke.

11 Clean up the hairline with a warm, moist towel. Apply astringent, moisturizing cream, talc, or after-shave lotion as desired.

CLEAN-UP AND DISINFECTION

☐ Clean and disinfect the tools and implements.
☐ Clean and then disinfect the work area.
☐ Sweep up hair and deposit in closed receptacle.
☐ Deposit used blades in a sharps container.
☐ Dispose of single-use items. Place all used linens, towels, and capes in the laundry.
☐ Wash your hands.

MILADY STANDARD SHAVING 61

P-11

THE HEAD SHAVE

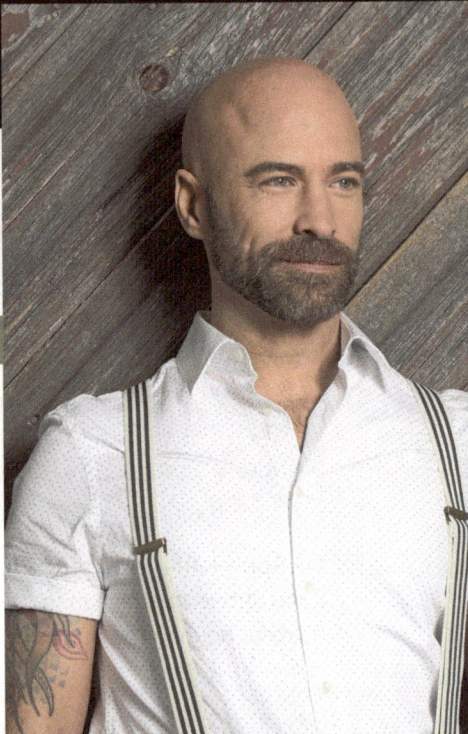

MATERIALS, IMPLEMENTS, AND EQUIPMENT

- ☐ All-purpose, taper, and flat top combs, picks, etc.
- ☐ Clipper disinfectant and coolant
- ☐ Clippers and outliners
- ☐ Disposable towels
- ☐ Hand mirror
- ☐ Neck strips
- ☐ Shampoo and conditioner
- ☐ Shampoo cape and haircutting cape
- ☐ Shaving cream or gel
- ☐ Spray bottle with water
- ☐ Straight razor and blades
- ☐ Talc
- ☐ Terry cloth towels
- ☐ Witch hazel or skin toner

PREPARATION

1. Wash your hands.
2. Conduct a client consultation.
3. Drape the client for a haircut.
4. Face the client toward the mirror and lock the chair.

PROCEDURE

1. Examine the scalp for any abrasions, primary or secondary lesions, or scalp disorders.

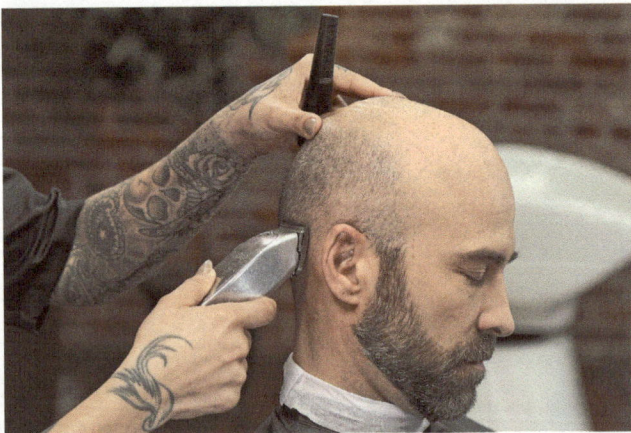

2. Remove excess hair length with the clippers if necessary; enough hair needs to remain for the razor to remove it without injuring the surface of the scalp.

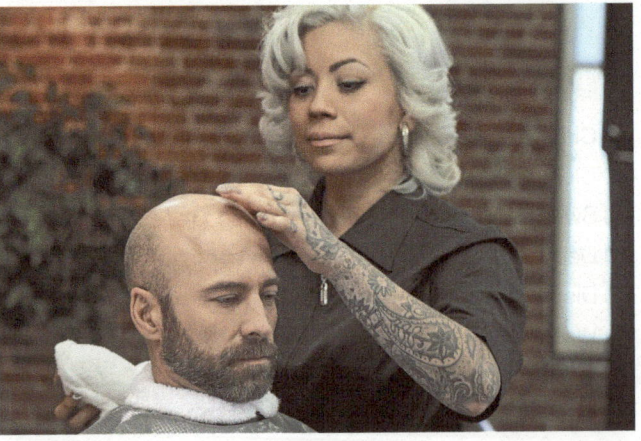

3. Drape the client for a wet service and shampoo the remaining hair; reexamine the scalp.

4. Remove the shampoo cape. Re-drape the client with a haircutting cape and towels under and over the drape. Tuck a wiping cloth into the neckline of the drape.

62 MILADY STANDARD SHAVING

PROCEDURE 11

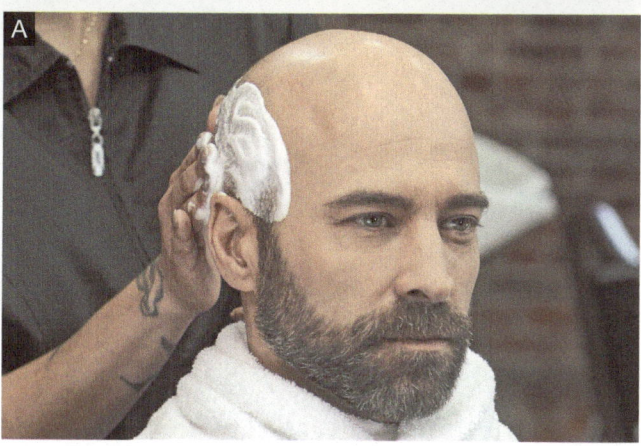 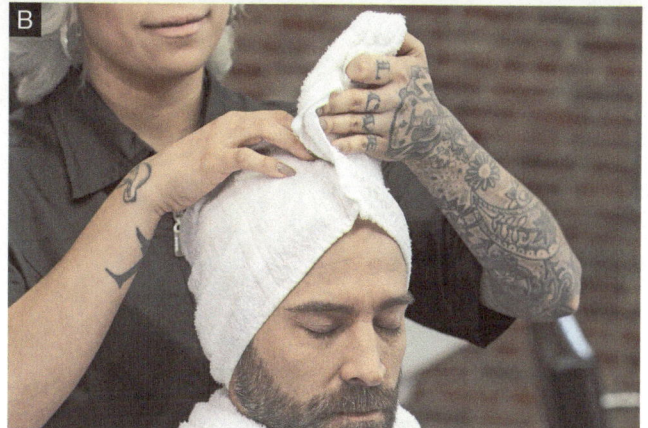

5️⃣ Apply shaving cream or gel and lather. Follow with two or three steamed-towel treatments to soften the remaining hair.

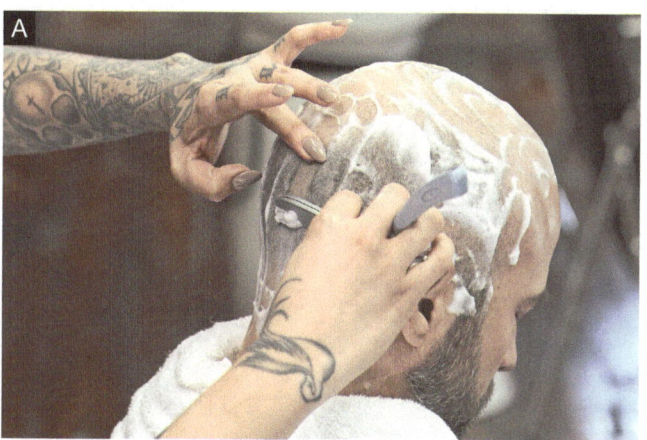 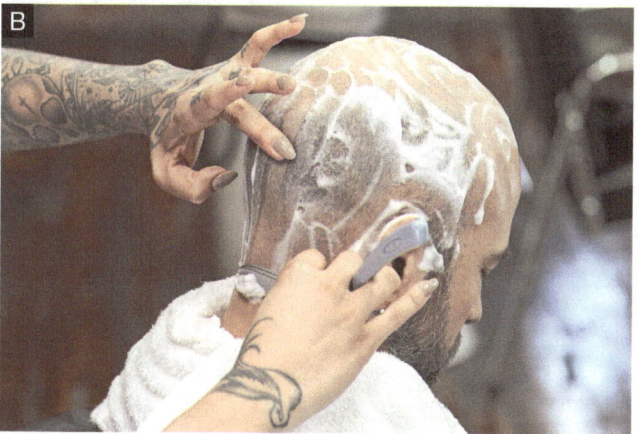

6️⃣ Re-lather the client's scalp and lock the chair. Start in the back section using a freehand stroke to shave with the grain of the hair from the crown to the nape. Use your opposite hand to stretch the skin taut as needed for each area to be shaved. Follow the curve of the head as you shave the entire back section.

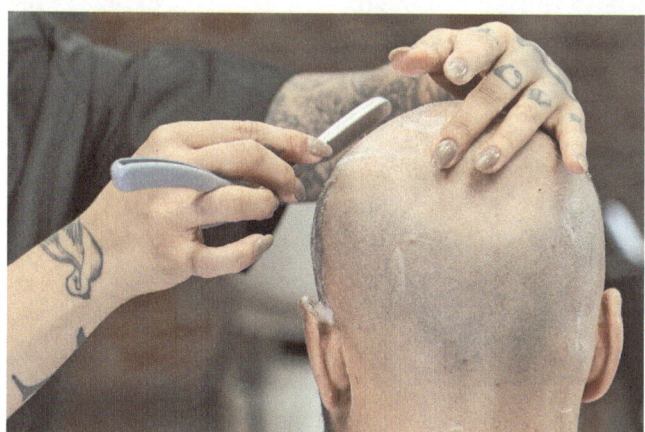

7️⃣ Move in front of the client and tip his head forward slightly. Continue shaving from the crown to the front hairline, reapplying lathering agent as needed. Remember to keep the skin moist to facilitate shaving.

MILADY STANDARD SHAVING   63

PROCEDURE 11

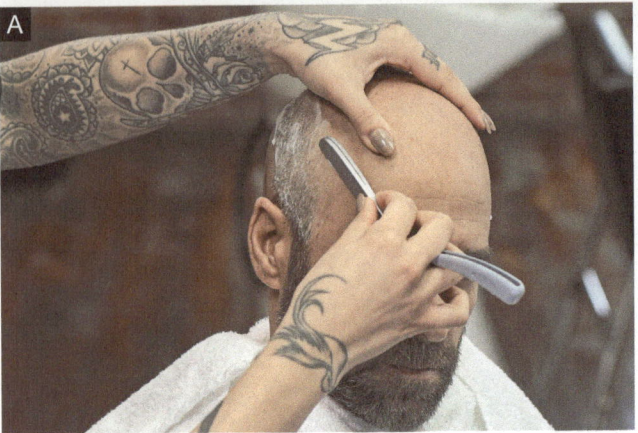
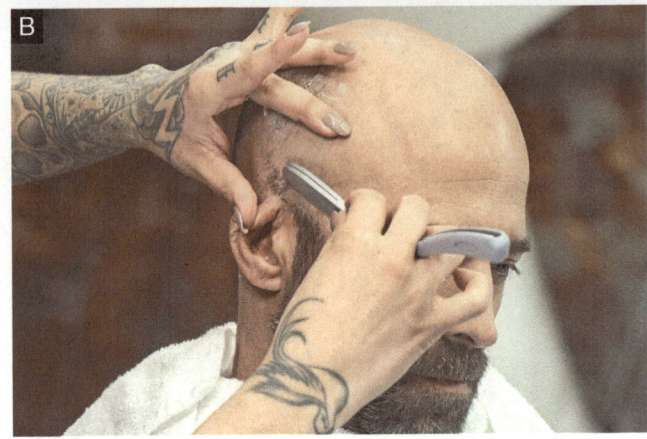

8 When the top section is completed, work down the sides. Just below the crest, hold the ear out of the way with the left hand, finish shaving the side, and carefully shave in front of and around the ears.

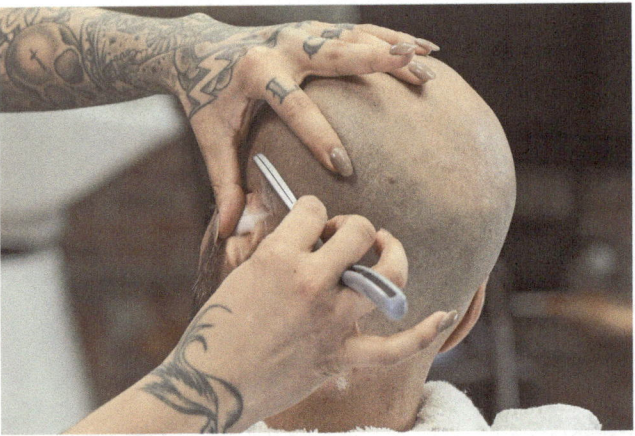
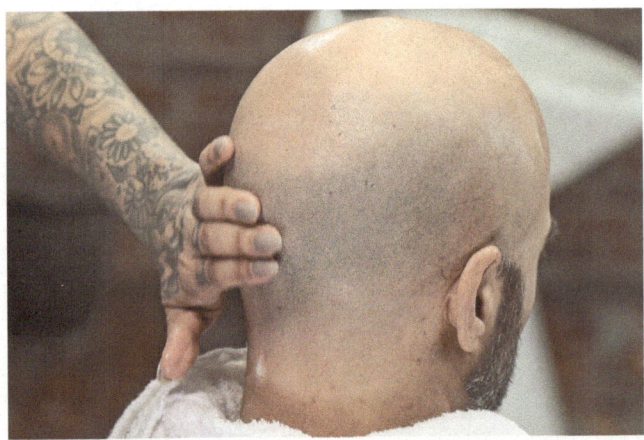

9 Repeat the shaving procedure on client's left side.

10 Check for any missed areas and re-shave as necessary.

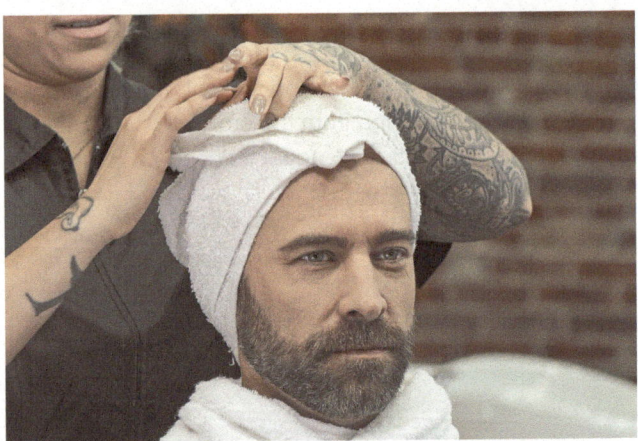
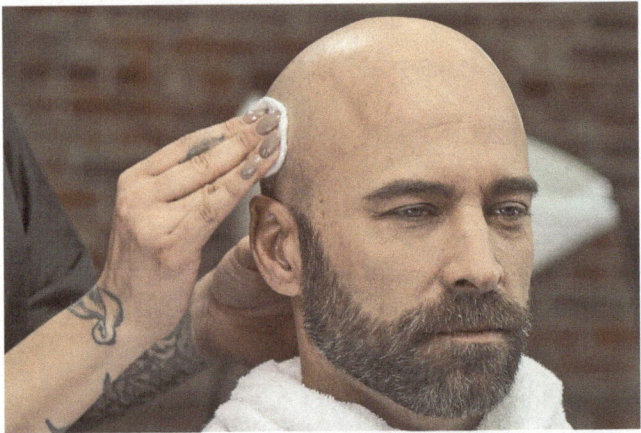

11 Wrap a warm towel around the client's head; then use it to remove any remaining lather.

12 Apply witch hazel or skin toner, and follow with a cool-towel application for 2 to 3 minutes.

PROCEDURE 11

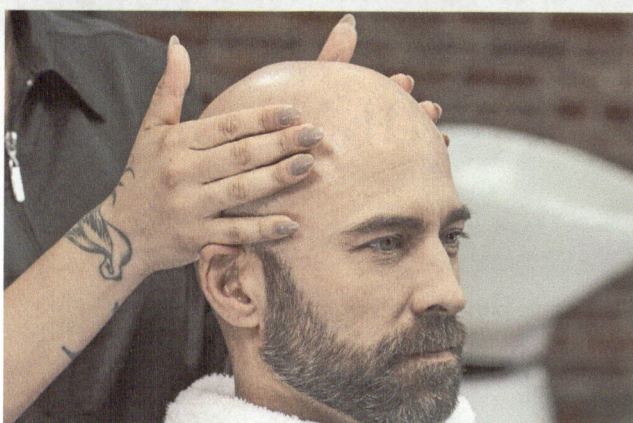

⑬ Apply moisturizing cream or oil as requested.

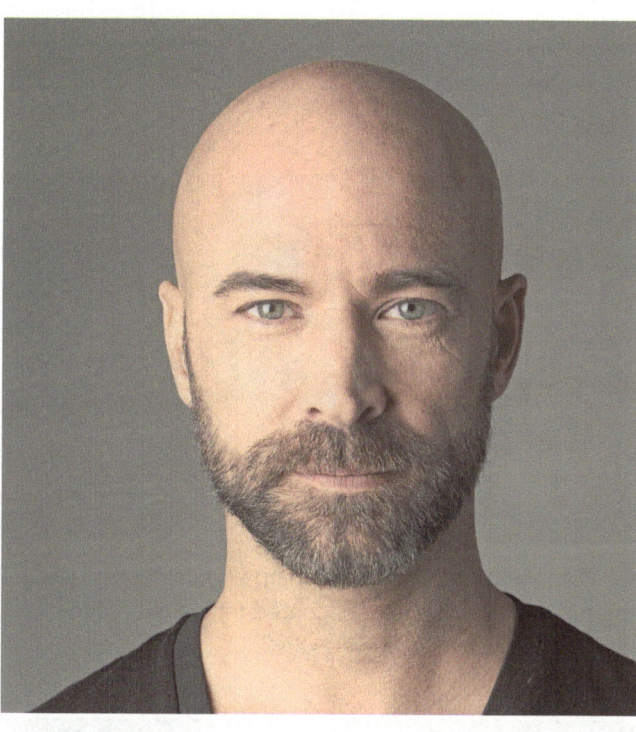

⑭ Finished head shave.

CLEAN-UP AND DISINFECTION

☐ Clean and disinfect the tools and implements.
☐ Clean and then disinfect the work area.
☐ Sweep up hair and deposit in a closed receptacle.
☐ Deposit used blades in a sharps container.
☐ Dispose of single-use items. Place all used linens, towels, and capes in the laundry.
☐ Wash your hands.

P-12

HANDLING AN EXPOSURE INCIDENT

MATERIALS, IMPLEMENTS, AND EQUIPMENT

- ☐ Antiseptic
- ☐ Bandages
- ☐ Cotton
- ☐ Disposable gloves
- ☐ Disposable paper towels
- ☐ Liquid soap
- ☐ Plastic bag

PROCEDURE

Should you accidentally cut a client, calmly take the following steps:

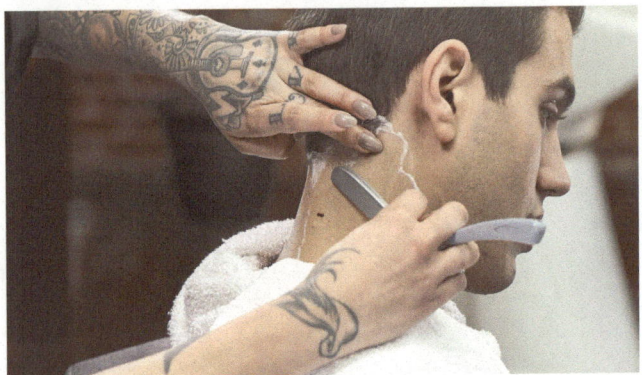

1 Stop the service immediately.

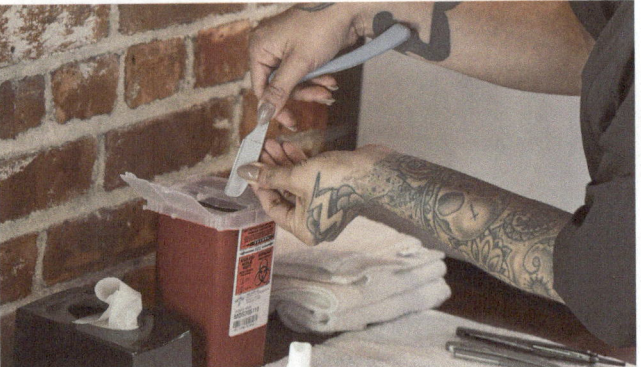

2 Dispose of the blade in a sharps container and place the razor in a container designated for cleaning and disinfection.

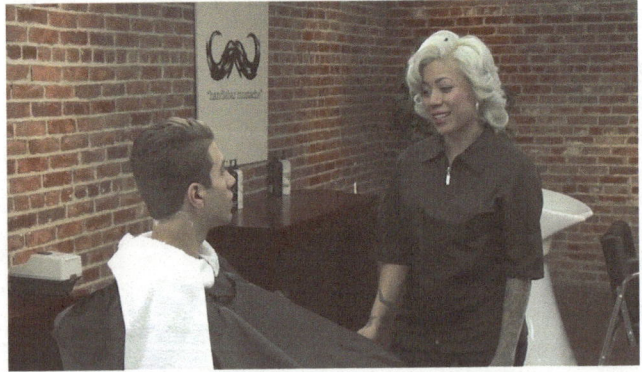

3 Face your client and calmly apologize for the incident.

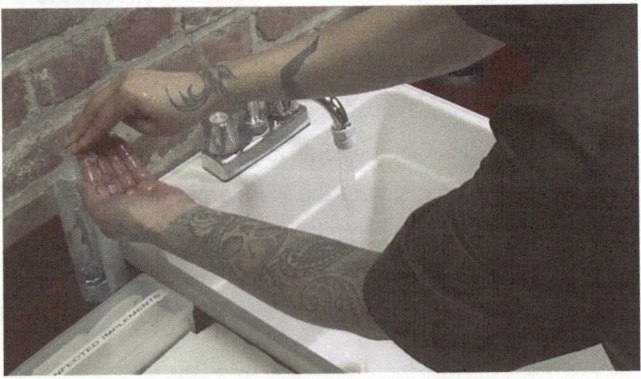

4 Excuse yourself to go wash your hands.

PROCEDURE 12

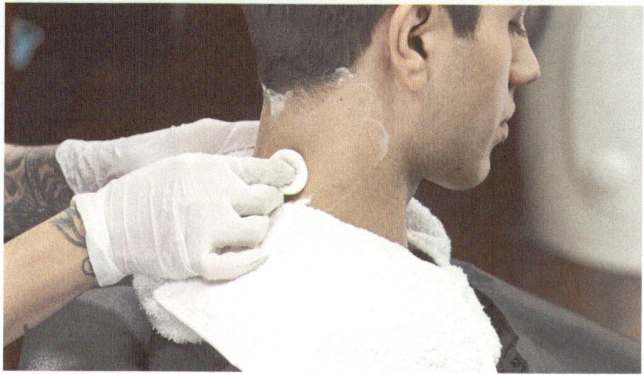

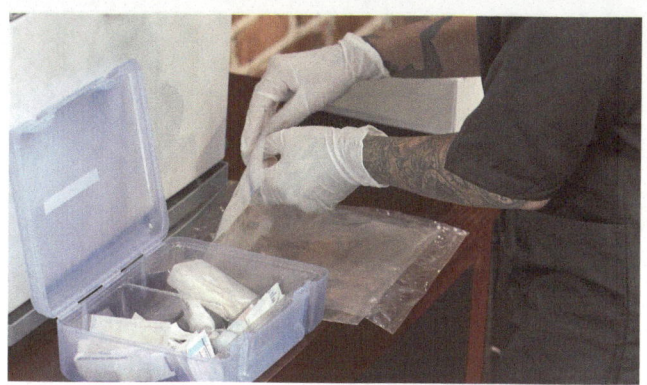

5 Once your hands are clean, immediately put on gloves.

6 Apply slight pressure to the area with a moistened cotton round to stop the bleeding.

7 Dispose of the used cotton round in a plastic storage bag.

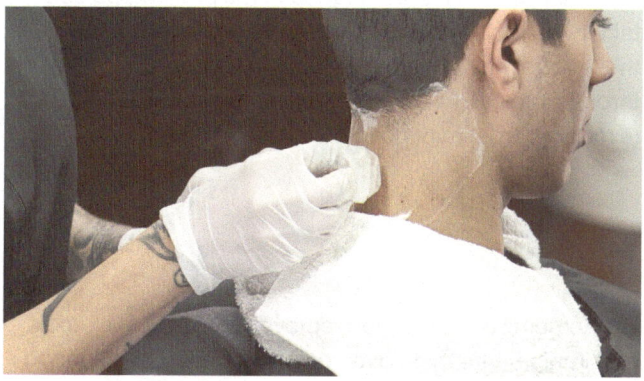

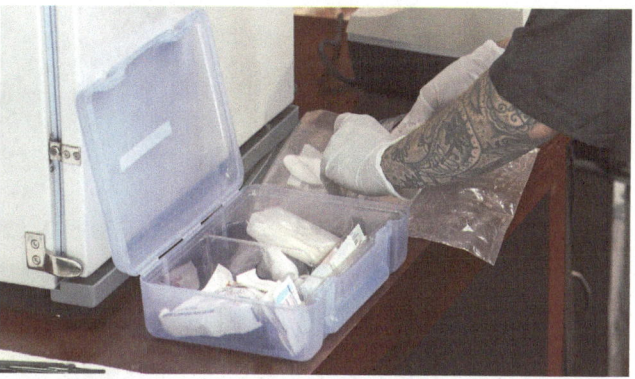

8 Then gently clean with an antiseptic and have the client wash the area if appropriate.

9 Dispose of the antiseptic wipe in the plastic storage bag.

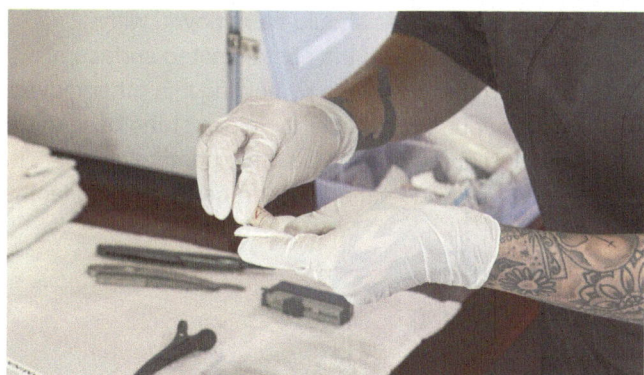

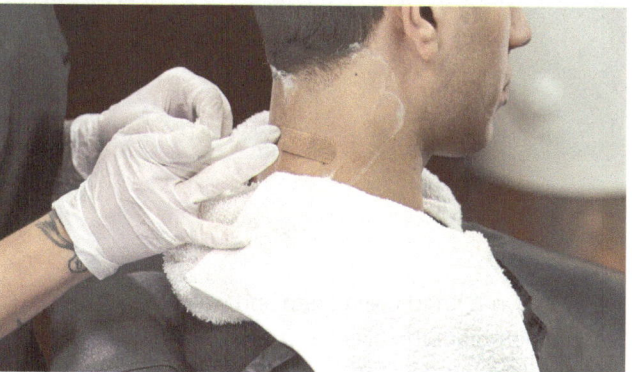

10 Dispense styptic powder onto a cotton round and use a cotton swab to apply it to the injury to stop any residual bleeding.

11 Apply an adhesive bandage to completely cover the wound.

MILADY STANDARD SHAVING

PROCEDURE 12

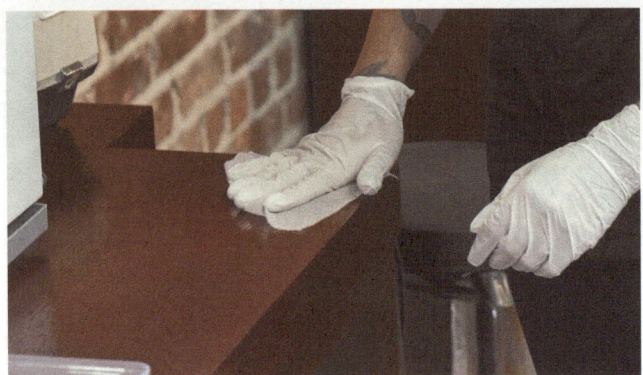

⑫ Clean and disinfect the workstation, as necessary.

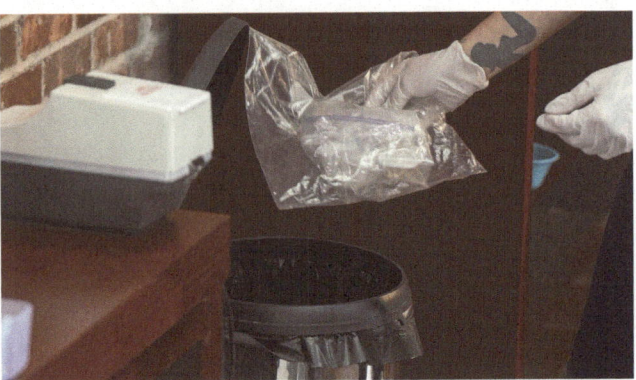

⑬ Discard all single-use, contaminated objects such as wipes or cotton balls in a plastic bag and then place in a trash bag. Deposit sharp disposables in a sharps box. Dispose of double-bagged items and sharps containers as required by state or local law. Information on these laws may be found on your local board website or through the OSHA website. In general, all of these items (except sharps) may go into the regular trash.

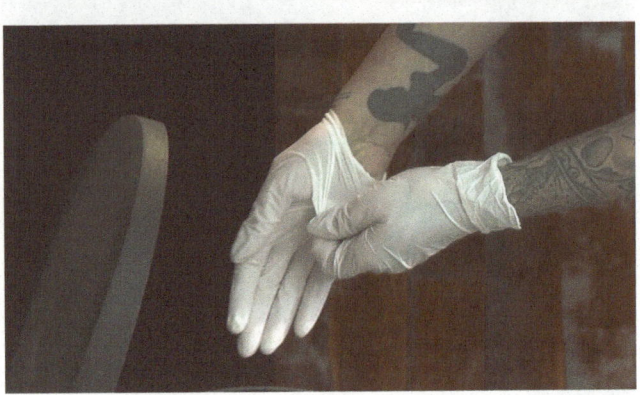

⑭ Remember, before you remove your gloves, all tools and implements that have come into contact with blood or other body fluids must be thoroughly cleaned and completely immersed in an EPA-registered hospital disinfectant solution designed for 10 minutes. Blood may carry pathogens, so you should never touch an open sore or a wound. Gloves should be removed with caution to avoid touching the contaminated surface of the glove. Remove one glove by holding it in other gloved hand, sliding your finger under the glove at the base of the glove, and pulling it over the other contaminated glove—never allowing either glove to come into contact with your skin.

⑮ Wash your hands with soap and warm water before returning to the service. Recommend that the client see a physician if any signs of redness, swelling, pain, or irritation develop.

REVIEW QUESTIONS

1. Name two types of straight razors.
2. List the basic parts of a straight razor.
3. Explain the purpose of a hone.
4. List three types of hones.
5. Explain the first and second positions and strokes used to hone a razor.
6. Explain the purpose of a strop.
7. What type of strop is considered the best for stropping a conventional straight razor?
8. Explain the first and second strokes used to strop a razor.
9. Identify three client characteristics that students should be aware of before beginning the shave service.
10. List the steps to prepare the client for a shave.
11. What effect does shaving cream have on facial hair?
12. Describe how to work shaving cream into a lather.
13. What effect do hot towels have on facial hair?
14. Identify several skin conditions that may prohibit the application of hot steam towels.
15. Identify the four razor-holding positions or strokes.
16. What three razor strokes are used in facial shaving?
17. Shaving strokes should be performed in what relation to the grain of the hair?
18. Identify the number of shaving areas of the face.
19. What two types of shaves are performed in a standard shave service?
20. Explain the difference between the first-time-over shave and the once-over shave.
21. List the finishing steps of a facial shave.
22. Explain how a close shave differs from a standard shave and why it may be undesirable.
23. List the important characteristics used to determine a mustache design.
24. Explain why some professionals prefer to cut and style the hair before performing a beard trim service.

GLOSSARY

backhand (BAK-HAND)	p. 14	razor position and stroke used in 4 of the 14 basic shaving areas: nos. 2, 6, 7, and 9; optional position for area 12
close shaving (KLOHS SHAYV-ing)	p. 21	the procedure of shaving facial hair against the grain during the second-time-over shave
cutting stroke (KUT-ing STROHK)	p. 14	the correct angle of cutting the beard with a straight razor
first-time-over shave (FIRST-TYM-OH-ver SHAYV)	p. 20	first part of the standard shave consisting of shaving the 14 areas of the face; followed by the second-time-over shave to remove residual missed or rough spots
freehand (FREE-HAND)	p. 14	razor position and stroke used in 6 of the 14 shaving areas: nos. 1, 3, 4, 8, 11, and 12
neck shave (NEK SHAYV)	p. 21	shaving the areas behind the ears down the sides of the neck, and at the back neckline
once-over shave (WONCE-OH-ver SHAYV)	p. 21	single-lather shave in which the shaving strokes are made across the grain of the hair
reverse backhand (ree-VURS BAK-HAND)	p. 14	razor position and stroke used by right-handed professionals for shaving the left side of the neck behind the ear and used by left-handed professionals behind the right ear
reverse freehand (ree-VURS FREE-HAND)	p. 14	razor position and stroke used in 4 of the 14 basic shaving areas: nos. 5, 10, 13, and 14
second-time-over shave (SEK-und-TYM-OH-ver SHAYV)	p. 20	follows a regular shave to remove any rough or uneven spots using water instead of lather; may be considered a form of close shaving
styptic powder (STIP-tik POW-dur)	p. 24	alum powder or liquid used to stop bleeding of nicks and cuts

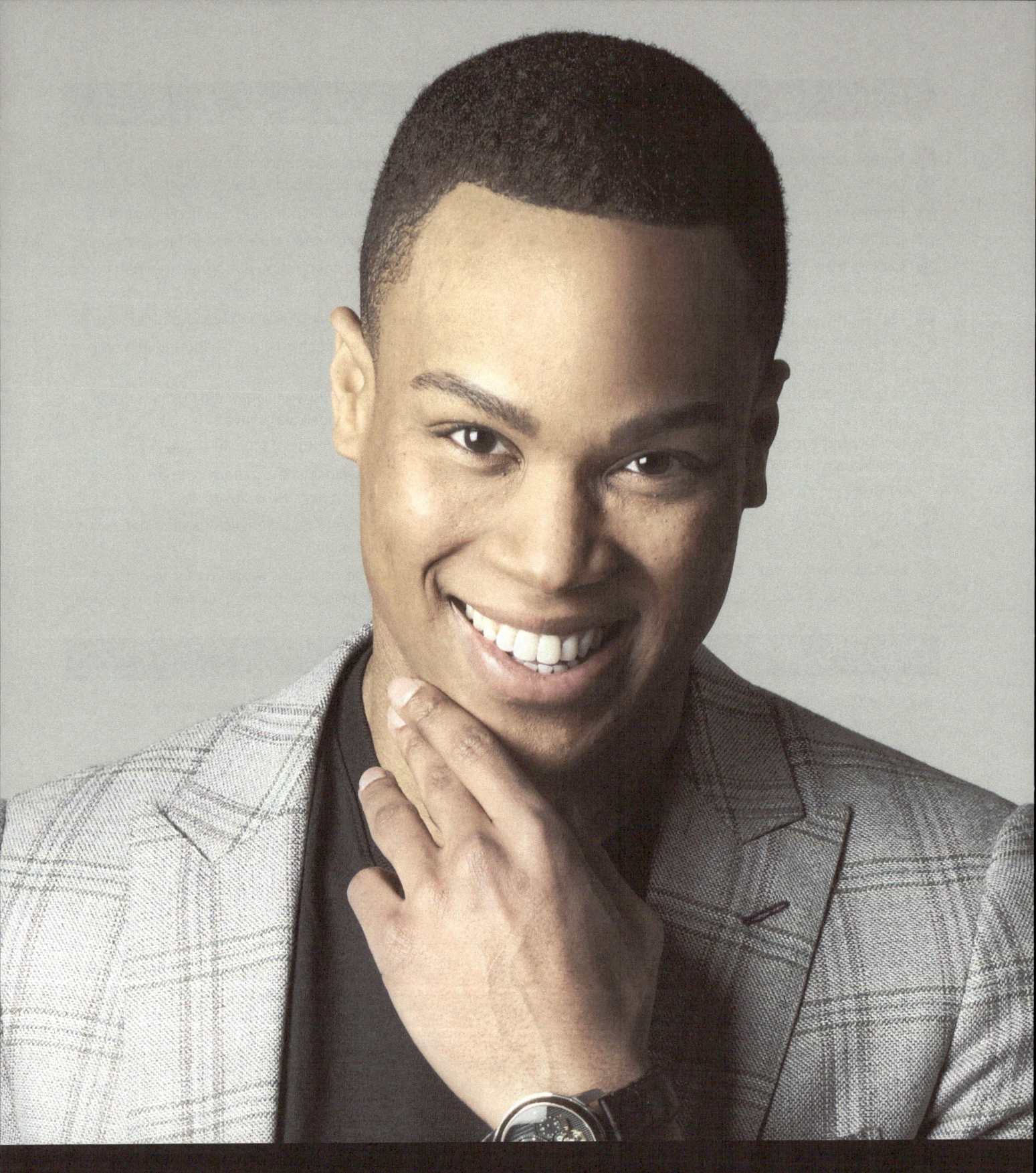

ACTIVITIES & TEST PREPARATION

ACTIVITIES

Know about Straight Razors

LO 1 Name two types of straight razors.

LO 2 Identify the different parts of a straight razor.

Fill-in-the-Blank

1 There are two types of straight razors: the _____ straight razor and the _____ straight razor.

Identify the Parts of a Straight Razor

Labeling

2 Label the parts of the razor in the following illustration.

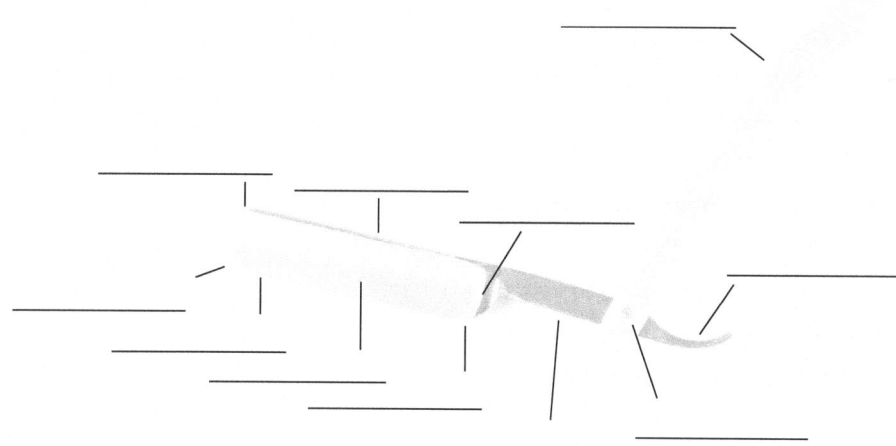

Show How to Hold a Straight Razor

LO 3 Show how to hold a straight razor for shaving, honing, and stropping.

LO 4 Show how to hold a straight razor for haircutting.

LO 5 Describe the functions of hones and strops.

LO 6 Show how to hone and strop a conventional blade straight razor.

Holding the Straight Razor

Fill-in-the-Blank

3 For shaving, the ball of the _____ and first two fingers are positioned on the _____ side of the shanks with the handle pivoted _____ to allow the little finger to rest on the _____.

4 For honing and stropping, the ball of the _____ and first two fingers are positioned on the _____ sides of the shank with the handle in a _____ position.

5 For haircutting, the ball of the _____ supports the razor at the bottom of the _____ and the little finger rests on the tang, with the first two or three fingers at the top of the _____.

Learn about Conventional Straight Razors

Fill-in-the-Blank

6 Razor _____ refers to the weight and length of the blade relative to that of the handle.

7 Razor _____ refers to the degree of hardness required for a good cutting edge, received from a special heat treatment during manufacturing.

8 The _____ of a razor is the shape of the blade after it has been ground. There are two general types: _____ and _____.

Hones and Strops

Matching

9 Match the following definitions with the most correct word or words.

_____ Removes any metal burrs or imbrications that remain after honing

_____ All-in-one accessory for preparing the razor after honing

_____ Produces a fine, long-lasting edge when used with water or shaving lather

_____ Produces a keen cutting edge in less time and may be used wet or dry

_____ Develops a good cutting edge and a fine finished edge

a. Natural hone
b. Synthetic hone
c. Canvas strop
d. Combination strop
e. Combination hone

Shaving and Facial-Hair Design

Short Answer/Fill-in-the-Blank

10 In your opinion, what are the benefits for men to have a professional shave over shaving at home?

_____
_____
_____
_____
_____
_____
_____

11 When performed correctly, a full facial shave, complete with _____, _____, and _____, is one of the most relaxing, yet rejuvenating, services men can enjoy.

Understand the Fundamentals of Shaving

LO 7   List basic guidelines for shaving a client.

LO 8   Identify the 14 shaving areas of the face.

LO 9   Explain what you need to know about razor positions and strokes to perform a shave safely and effectively.

Consider Basic Guidelines for Shaving a Client

Fill-in-the-Blank/Case Study

12 Do not proceed with the service if the client has a _____ or _____.

13 _____ the client's hair growth pattern before beginning the shave to identify grain changes and growth patterns in the beard.

14 Do not use _____ on skin that is chapped, blistered, thin, or sensitive.

15 Do not perform a(n) _____ immediately after a shave as it may irritate or damage the skin.

16 Use _____ fresheners or _____ when stronger astringents are too harsh for sensitive skin.

17 When a client wears a _____, trim and shape it prior to the shave service to prepare it for finish work with the razor during the shave.

18 Be careful when shaving sensitive areas beneath the _____, on the lower part of the _____, and around the Adam's apple to avoid irritation or injury.

19 **Knowing When Not to Shave**

A shave service has many benefits for the client, such as relaxation. However, there are times when a client must be declined for a shave service. Identify one or two instances in which you would have to tell a client that a shave cannot be performed and explain why. Explain what you would do instead.

_____

_____

_____

_____

_____

_____

_____

Identifying the Shaving Areas of the Face

Labeling

20 Number the shaving areas in the following illustration depending on whether you are right-handed or left-handed. Next, draw the directional arrows for each area.

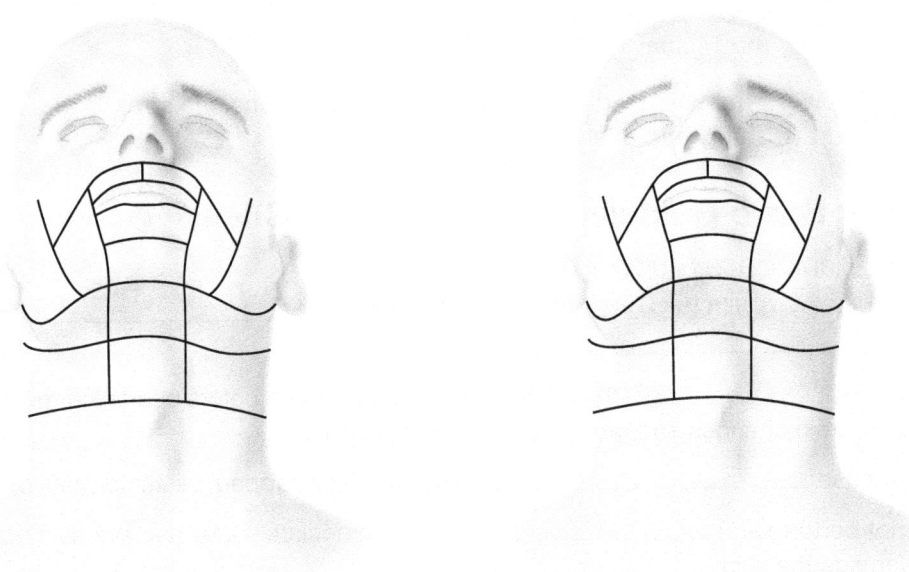

Understand Razor Positions and Strokes

Fill-in-the-Blank

21 To achieve a proper cutting stroke, the razor is positioned at a slight _____ to the skin surface and stroked with the point _____.

22 The three positions and strokes used in facial shaving are _____, _____, and _____.

23 _____ refers to the way the razor is held in the professional's hand to perform a stroke movement.

24 It is important to know how to position the fingers, wrist, and elbow of the _____ hand in relation to the razor.

25 A professional must know how to use the _____ and _____ finger as the primary digits for stretching the skin.

26 A professional must angle the razor about _____ degrees relative to the skin surface.

Handling a Straight Razor

Fill-in-the-Blank

27 To open the razor, grasp the _____ of the blade between the _____ and index finger of the dominant hand while holding the handle with the opposite thumb and index finger.

28 Hold the razor between the thumb and index finger on the sides of the _____ near the shoulder of the blade and rest across the _____ and third fingers, with the _____ finger bracing the razor.

29 When closing the razor, release the _____ finger and bring the _____ to the blade.

Razor Position and Strokes Practice

Matching/Short Answer/Fill-in-the-Blank

30 Match the descriptions with the correct razor position and stroke.

   _____ Handle of razor should rest between the third and fourth fingers

   _____ Underside of handle rests on the third and fourth fingers

   _____ Left hand should be positioned above the razor

   _____ Razor edge should be turned upward

   a. Freehand
   b. Backhand
   c. Reverse-freehand
   d. Reverse-backhand

31 List the shaving areas in which the freehand position and stroke is used.

   • _____
   • _____
   • _____
   • _____
   • _____

32 Explain when the reverse backhand stroke may be used.

   _____
   _____

33 List the shaving areas in which the backhand stroke is used.

- _____
- _____
- _____
- _____
- _____

34 With the reverse-backhand position and stroke, use a smooth, _____ stroke, directed _____ that leads with the point of the razor.

35 With the reverse-freehand position and stroke, use a(n) _____, semi-arced stroke toward you with the point leading in a _____ movement.

36 With the freehand stroke, _____ with the point of the razor in a _____, gliding movement.

Understand Body Positioning

Fill-in-the-Blank

37 If you are a right-handed student, you will stand at the client's _____ side.

38 If you are a left-handed student, you will stand at the client's _____ side.

39 To change position, take _____ steps or shift your body weight from one _____ to the other.

Describe the Professional Shave

Multiple Choice

40 The skin is held _____ to create the correct shaving surface for the razor.

- a. tightly
- c. firmly
- b. loosely
- d. not at all

41 When shaving a client, excess lather should be removed with the _____

- a. thumb
- c. index finger
- b. forefinger
- d. pinky finger

42 _____ skin allows the beard hair to be cut more easily.

- a. Dry
- c. Bumpy
- b. Loose
- d. Taut

Know the Types of Shaves

Fill-in-the-Blank/Short Answer/Multiple Choice

43 A(n) _____ shave should ensure a complete and even shave with a single lathering.

44 _____ is the practice of shaving the beard against the grain during the second-time-over phase of the shave.

45 With the second-time-over shave, the client's skin is moistened with a(n) _____ towel or water and a(n) _____ stroke is used to shave with or across the grain to remove any remaining hair.

46 Describe the difference between a traditional neck shave and an outline shave.

_____
_____
_____
_____
_____
_____
_____

47 Which part of the head and neck is *not* shaved during a traditional neck shave?

    a. Behind the ears.   c. Both sides of the neck.

    b. Across the nape.   d. Front hairline.

Understand Facial-Hair Design: Mustaches

LO 10 Describe the differences between various facial hair designs.

Multiple Choice/Matching

48 Which of the following characteristics of facial features does *not* influence mustache design?

    a. Size of the nose.   c. Size of the eyes.

    b. Shape of upper lip area.   d. Width of the mouth.

49 Match the facial features with the appropriate mustache design.

___ Long, narrow face

___ Extra-small mouth

___ Round face with regular features

___ Square face with prominent features

___ Extra-large mouth

___ Prominent nose

___ Large, coarse facial features

___ Wide mouth with prominent upper lip

___ Smallish, regular features

a. Heavier-looking mustache

b. Medium to large mustache

c. Narrow to medium mustache

d. Pyramid-shaped mustache

e. Medium, short mustache

f. Smaller, triangular mustache

g. Heavier handlebar or large divided mustache

h. Semi-square mustache

i. Heavier, linear mustache with ends slightly curving downward

Designing the Beard

Fill-in-the-Blank

50 Analyze the _____ and _____ of the hair to identify uneven growth areas.

51 Consider where hair growth under the _____ and _____ changes direction to help determine design options for outlines in this area.

52 Leave the facial hair slightly _____ than the desired end result during the _____ trimming to avoid cutting the hair too closely.

53 _____ clipper-cutting is most successful on beards with even density and texture.

54 Beard trimming and design is usually performed with a combination of the _____, _____, outliner and/or clippers, and razor.

Review Shaving-Related Infection Control and Safety Precautions

LO 11   Discuss infection control and safety precautions associated with shaving.

Fill-in-the-Blank

55 _____ and _____ razors and blades before use.

56 _____ used blades in a sharps container.

57 Wash your hands _____ servicing a client.

58 Use _____ linens, capes, and paper products.

59 Provide a clean cloth or paper barrier between the client's head and the _____.

60 Treat small cuts or nicks using standard precautions and _____ procedures.

61 _____ the chair once the client is properly draped and in position for the shave.

62 Prepare _____ hair for the shave with warm or hot towels and lather.

63 Use a light touch and a forward _____ motion that leads with the point of the blade.

64 Observe the _____ and shave with it, not against it.

65 _____ against the grain gently to place the hair in a position to be shaved.

66 Keep your fingers _____ to stretch or hold the skin firmly during the shave.

67 Use the cushions of the fingertips to stretch skin in the _____ direction of the razor stroke.

68 Keep the fingers and thumb of the _____ hand away from the path of the razor.

69 Apply _____ neatly to the areas to be shaved and replace as necessary.

70 Keep the skin _____ while shaving.

71 Follow through with shaving strokes from one shaving area to another; do not stop _____ or shave over an area repeatedly.

Word Review

Fill-in-the-Blank

Backhand	Neck shave	Second-time-over shave
Cutting stroke	Once-over shave	Styptic powder
First-time-over shave	Reverse backhand	
Freehand	Reverse freehand	

MILADY STANDARD SHAVING

_____: Alum powder or liquid used to stop bleeding of nicks and cuts.

_____: Razor position and stroke used in 4 of the 14 basic shaving areas: nos. 2, 6, 7, and 9; optional position for area 12.

_____: A single-lather shave in which the shaving strokes are made across the grain of the hair.

_____: A razor position and stroke used in 4 of the 14 basic shaving areas: nos. 5, 10, 13, and 14.

_____: The first part of the standard shave consisting of shaving the 14 areas of the face; followed by the second-time-over shave to remove residual missed or rough spots.

_____: A shaving technique that follows a regular shave to remove any rough or uneven spots using water instead of lather; may be considered a form of close shaving.

_____: Razor position and stroke used in 6 of the 14 shaving areas: nos. 1, 3, 4, 8, 11, and 12.

_____: The correct angle of cutting the beard with a straight razor.

_____: Shaving the areas behind the ears down the sides of the neck, and at the back neckline.

_____: A razor position and stroke used by right-handed professionals for shaving the left side of the neck behind the ear and used by left-handed professionals behind the right ear.

TEST PREPARATION

Multiple Choice

1. What is the razor of choice for professional shaving?
   - a. Trimmer.
   - b. Straight.
   - c. Safety.
   - d. Edger.

2. You should avoid judging a razor simply on _____.
   - a. color or design
   - b. quality
   - c. other professional's recommendations
   - d. manufacturer

3. What type of razor tends to be used almost exclusively in the professional settings because it helps to maintain infection control standards?
   - a. Hair shaper.
   - b. Conventional straight razor.
   - c. Changeable-blade straight razor.
   - d. Razor shaper.

4. The method for replacing the blade in a changeable-razor will vary depending on the _____.
   - a. model
   - b. procedure
   - c. shave
   - d. holding technique

5. If the razor handle is in a straightened position with the thumb and first two fingers almost touching at the shank, this is the technique for _____.
   - a. stropping
   - b. honing
   - c. shaving
   - d. haircutting

6. If the ball of the thumb and first two fingers are positioned on the flat side of the shanks with the handle pivoted up to allow the little finger to rest on the tang, this is the technique for_____.
   - a. shaving
   - b. honing
   - c. haircutting
   - d. stropping

7. Which of the following positions gives the most control of the razor when honing and stropping?
   - a. The ball of the thumb supports the razor at the bottom of the shank and the little finger rests on the tang with the first two or three fingers at the top of the shank.
   - b. The ball of the thumb and first two fingers are positioned on the flat side of the shanks with the handle pivoted up to allow the little finger to rest on the tang.
   - c. The ball of the thumb and first two fingers are positioned on the flat sides of the shank with the handle in a straight position.
   - d. The razor handle is in a straightened position with the thumb and first two fingers almost touching at the shank.

8. When a razor is properly _____, it acquires the degree of hardness required for a good cutting edge.
   a. finished
   b. balanced
   c. tempered
   d. sized

9. Which of the following refers to the weight and length of the blade relative to that of the handle?
   a. Razor size.
   b. Razor grind.
   c. Razor temper.
   d. Razor balance.

10. What is used to grind the steel and impart an effective cutting edge to the razor's blade?
    a. Temper.
    b. Strop.
    c. Hone.
    d. Grind.

11. A keen razor edge has fine teeth and tends to dig into a thumbnail _____.
    a. without any cutting power
    b. with a smooth, steady grip
    c. with a jerky feeling
    d. with a harsh, grating sound

12. The direction of the blade edge in stropping is the reverse of that used in _____.
    a. honing
    b. stroking
    c. bracing
    d. edging

13. What pace is preferred when stropping?
    a. Slow.
    b. Uneven.
    c. Fast.
    d. Moderate.

14. Which of the following will you not perform immediately after a shave?
    a. Second-time-over shave.
    b. Deep cleansing facial.
    c. Applying fresheners or toners.
    d. Applying a warm towel.

15. The application of _____ is a standard procedure in preparing the beard for shaving.
    a. toners
    b. fresheners
    c. hot towels
    d. astringents

16. Do not proceed with the shave service if the client has _____.
    a. pustules
    b. whorl growth patterns
    c. chapped skin
    d. a keloid condition

17. What determines hairline shapes?
    a. Skin type.
    b. Facial-hair design.
    c. Hair texture.
    d. Growth patterns.

18. _____ are often the result of improper hair removal by a razor, tweezers, or trimmer.
    a. Pustules
    b. Skin infections
    c. Ingrown hairs
    d. Whorls

19. Do not use hot towels on skin that is _____.
    a. tanned
    b. chapped
    c. wrinkled
    d. freckled

20. Be careful when shaving sensitive areas such as _____.
    a. around the Adam's apple
    b. on the cheekbones
    c. upper part of the neck
    d. on top of the lip

21. When a client wears a mustache, trim and shape it _____ the shave service.
    a. closer than
    b. after
    c. during
    d. prior to

22. Ingrown hairs are also known as _____.
    a. pustules
    b. folliculitis
    c. pseudofolliculitis
    d. a keloid condition

23. Which of the following is a reason a client may find fault with a shave procedure?
    a. Warm fingers.
    b. Heavy touch.
    c. Sharp razors.
    d. Soft overhead lights.

24. There are 14 shaving areas of the face to be shaved during the _____ part of the service.
    a. close shave
    b. second-time-over
    c. first-time-over
    d. once-over shave

25. The 14 shaving areas of the face are shaved _____ and sequentially from one section to another.
    a. quickly
    b. repeatedly
    c. diagonally
    d. systematically

26. During the first-time-over part of the service, you would shave _____ in each of the 14 areas of the face.
    a. with the grain
    b. against the grain
    c. across the grain
    d. in a circular manner

27. The shaving movement from the angle of mouth toward point of chin would be which of the following?
    a. Freehand and down.
    b. Backhand and down.
    c. Reverse freehand and up.
    d. Freehand and across.

28. The shaving movement from beneath the lower lip would be _____.
    a. backhand and down
    b. freehand and down
    c. reverse freehand and up
    d. backhand and down

29. What type of strokes do you use around the mouth, over the ears, and in other tight areas?
    a. Faster.
    b. Shorter.
    c. Medium.
    d. Longer.

30. Lathering with a shaving cream or gel _____.
    a. softens the hair cuticle
    b. provides lubrication by stimulating oil glands
    c. relaxes the client
    d. cleanses the skin

31. Stretching the skin too tightly will cause _____.
    a. nicks
    b. cuts
    c. irritation
    d. ingrown hairs

32. What type of shaving is the practice of shaving the beard against the grain during the second-time-over phase of the shave?
    a. Close.
    b. Once-over shave.
    c. Outline.
    d. Complete.

33. What type of shave should result in a smooth face without being a close shave?
    a. Outline.
    b. First-time-over.
    c. Second-time-over.
    d. Once-over shave.

34. For a man who has an extra-large mouth, what type of mustache would be complimentary?
    a. Heavier-looking.
    b. Pyramid-shaped.
    c. Semi-square.
    d. Medium to large.

35. Beards can be used to _____ the appearance of facial features.
    a. dominant
    b. minimize
    c. balance
    d. perfect

36. You should angle the razor how many degrees relative to the skin surface?
    a. 10 degrees.
    b. 30 degrees.
    c. 45 degrees.
    d. 90 degrees.

37. The correct angle of cutting with a razor is called the _____ stroke.
    a. cutting
    b. freehand
    c. gliding
    d. proper

38. Which of the following refers to the way the razor is held in the hand to perform a stroke movement?
    a. Angle.
    b. Grain.
    c. Position.
    d. Procedure.

39. You would apply light facial cream or moisturizing lotion with what type of movement?
    a. Pétrissage massage.
    b. Forward gliding.
    c. Sliding.
    d. Effleurage massage.

40. Right-handed professionals stand at the client's _____.
    a. right side
    b. back
    c. left side
    d. front

41. Which of the following is an antihemorrhagic?
    a. Alcohol.
    b. Astringent.
    c. Styptic powder.
    d. pH-balanced fresheners or toners.

42. What razor position and stroke is *not* used in facial shaving?
    a. Freehand.
    b. Reverse backhand.
    c. Backhand.
    d. Reverse freehand.

43. When performing a shave service, you would use the _____ to stretch the skin with the proper amount of pressure.
    a. cushions of the fingertips
    b. thumbs
    c. palms
    d. little fingers

44. The reverse-backhand stroke is only used during a _____ shave.
    a. once-over
    b. neck
    c. first-time-over
    d. second-time-over

45. Preparation includes which of the following?
    a. Light powder dusting.
    b. Toning.
    c. Draping the client.
    d. Massaging moisturizer into the skin.

46. Steaming helps to _____.
    a. hold the hair in an upright position
    b. cleanse the skin
    c. create a smooth surface for the razor
    d. provide lubrication by stimulating oil glands

47. What type of skin allows the beard hair to be cut more easily?
    a. Taut.
    b. Loose.
    c. Tight.
    d. Dry.

48. Which of the following shaves should ensure a complete and even shave with a single lathering?
    a. First-time-over.
    b. Close.
    c. Once-over shave.
    d. Second-time-over.

49. Be sure to check the hairline and neck areas for _____ before beginning the neck shave.
    a. rough or uneven spots
    b. hypertrophies
    c. taut skin
    d. ingrown hairs

50. _____ cutting is most successful on beards with even density and texture.
    a. Razor cutting
    b. Shear-over-comb
    c. Outliner-over-comb
    d. Even-all-over clipper

51. Following the first-time-over shave, the professional checks the client's skin for any _____.
    a. cuts
    b. hypertrophies
    c. rough or uneven spots
    d. nicks

52. Finishing a shave would include which of the following?
    a. Steaming the face.
    b. Massaging moisturizer into the skin.
    c. Stretching the skin.
    d. Lathering the face with cream or gel.

53. When performing a shave service, you should keep the nondominant thumb and fingertips dry for _____ purposes.
    a. stretching
    b. stroking
    c. positioning
    d. finishing

54. Do not stop short or shave over an area _____.
    a. systematically
    b. gently
    c. repeatedly
    d. sequentially

55. Keep your fingers _____ to stretch or hold the skin firmly during the shave.
    a. powdered
    b. dry
    c. gloved
    d. moist

56. When performing a shave, you would use a light touch and what type of motion that leads with the point of the blade?
    a. Very fast.
    b. Very slow.
    c. Sliding.
    d. Forward gliding.

57. Where should you discard used blades?
    a. Trash basket.
    b. Plastic garbage bag.
    c. Sharps container.
    d. Closed receptacle.

58. Keep the skin _____ while shaving.
    a. hot
    b. moist
    c. dry
    d. cold

59. Treat small cuts or nicks using standard precautions and _____ procedures.
    a. exposure incident
    b. first aid
    c. disinfectant
    d. safety

NOTES

NOTES

NOTES

NOTES

NOTES

NOTES